TOJIK-INDIAN YOGA
SECRETS

TOJIK-INDIAN YOGA SECRETS

HEALTH, HAPPINESS AND HARMONY ON EARTH

SOBIROV/MISHRA

PARTRIDGE

A Penguin Company

Partridge books may be ordered through booksellers or by contacting:

Partridge India
Penguin Books India Pvt.Ltd
11, Community Centre, Panchsheel Park, New Delhi 110017
India
www.partridgepublishing.com
Phone: 000.800.10062.62

CONTENTS

PART FOUR

The book has got four parts. The first one is basically autobiographical with a view to bring home the readers how Abduvahob Sobirov, a Muslim by birth gets so much engrossed in a system he would hardly find any support from his tradition. But Sobirov takes the readers much farther to suggest that the present divide caused by known history will no way affect the imminent fundamental unity of mankind which must usher in a short while from now.

Part Two imparts some of the important principles of Yoga teachings. Part Three is the India of Sobir's dream and aspiration. It also records India's thick relationship with him.

The Fourth part strongly urges that Yoga is now a Global Cult and it should undoubtedly unite all peoples on the earth to live in harmony and peace for ever.

In the appendix part Sobirov has reproduced some valuable information about the values of food stuff we take and should be aware of in our daily food habit.

Its editor and co-author PD Mishra evidently contributes substantially with a cross-border bond of unity (Yoga) by his intrinsic presence throughout.

INTRODUCTION

Practising Yoga since 1984 without a teacher, without books, simply travelling to India for confirmation of ideas 10 times, I've found that I'm one of the followers of Buddha generation. Many statues have been found in our country in yoga postures and one Buddha statue of 13 meters is exhibited now in Japan. I'm the president of Yoga Association in my country since 1990 and a director since 1985. I'm very strict and disciplined in Yogic philosophy and practice. I've published about 10 books and 150 articles in Tojik, Russian, English and Hindi so far. This long book is now in English with an intention of a global reach. The great secret of my life is that in 1986, after 3 years of individual practice in Yoga by books, my third eye was opened. There came a prediction for me that the USSR will disintegrate soon,—I'll tell about it in detail in pages to follow. Since that time I have become a fighter for a brighter life of Yoga. My past life of Yogic experiences has been a boon to me as I am curing all sorts of ailments through it.

The present book is written particularly in view of the readers of India, Tajikistan and the whole world in general for demonstrating the reality of Yoga. Dear readers, after reading this book, you will not regret why you have purchased it. You may have many books on yoga at your disposal, but the Yoga which cures every disease momentarily, just in one day, one week, one month and one year's prescription, is here. It depends on the seriousness of disease and the patient. I may not be one like many yogis & gurus of India & some other countries, but I'm one from you who has had a turning point like every one of you now must have. I am therefore, briefly recording my story of my life since my birth in high different coloured mountainous village of Tojikistan.

My life has been very complicated, curved, and difficult with mysteries unknown to me till now. P. D. Mishra was the only yogi who came to my country and opened my eyes to yoga inviting me to come to India. He took me around this great land showing the places of wonder. I am now completing this vibrating work in his company and care. He has already written a number of books on Yoga, philosophy, literature and Vedic science. We are confident that this book is received very warmly by all seekers of the truth around the world.

Dusanbey, Tojikistan   **Abduvahob Sobirov (Yogishwranand)**

MY SIDE OF IT

Abduvahob Sobirov wanted me to edit and co-author this book as it indeed comprises mostly his vista and vision of Yoga and India in his deep trust and conviction. He has already worked so hard in it that it became still harder for me to compress and compile it with the Indian audience in view in particular and the new dimensions of cross-border Yoga teachings throughout the world now.

It has got four parts. The first one is basically autobiographical with a view to bring home the readers how **Abduvahob Sobirov**, a Muslim by birth gets so much engrossed in a system he would hardly find any support from his tradition. But Sobirov takes the readers much farther to suggest that the present divide caused by known history will no way affect the imminent fundamental unity of mankind which must usher in a short while from now.

Part Two imparts some of the important principles of Yoga teachings. Part Three is the India of Sobir's dream and aspiration. It also well records India's thick relationship with him.

The Fourth part strongly urges that Yoga is now a Global Cult and it should undoubtedly unite all peoples on the globe to live in harmony and peace for ever.

In the appendix part Sobirov has reproduced valuable information about the values of food stuff we use and should certainly be aware of in our daily food.

I sincerely hope that the book is a great welcome in India and abroad.

P D. Mishra, President Maharshi Agastya Vedic Sansthanam, Bhopal, India

(www.vishwatm.com, email-pdmishra@operamail.com)

PART ONE

1

TOJIK YOGA

YOGA in Tajikistan now exists since 1986. It is a quite advanced system helping people of all ages for getting rid of many illnesses in a short span of time. I, A. SOBIROV, (now Yogishwranand) a Tojik by birth, am practicing it for over 27 years. My system has been approved widely especially in Russia, Byelorussia and in India. In Tajikistan now about one fifth of its population has faith in it and practices it. I am a total vegetarian, pure and quickly accessible welcoming individuals—needy ones. In order to prove how radically it changed my life, I am herein recording for sharing purposes some of the details and dilemmas of my life which themselves teach many lessons necessary in everyone's life to move in this direction of light, energy and happiness.

"Never put off till tomorrow what you can do today".

TOJIK BUDDHA

In the town Mandara (Japan) there was the ceremony of opening a new historical museum. In it now is exhibited a 13 meter long Tojik-Buddha statue which is 1300 years old. It came to be known to the Ministry of economy and trade of the country in 2005 only. The image of Tojik historical Buddha is one of the important exhibits in Tojik exposure in "EXPO—2005" in Ychi city of Japan. Millions of tourists, archaeologists and researchers to Japan have visited and seen it. Now the Tojik Buddha is exhibited in the new museum, the north city Nagoi—a place of the undertaking of "EXPO—2005".

BUDDHA IN AFGHANISTAN

As a historical evidence and archaeological support, it is worth recollection here that In Bomiyan (Afghanistan) there were statues of Buddha with the length of 55 meters. Taliban did not appreciate these historically valuable monuments and during one bloodthirsty war, they even destroyed them partially.

Why Buddha statues with such a vastness and length having great historical importance in the world were built in Afghanistan? And again in Tajikistan too? Why?

These questions have been haunting me ever since too much. I heard that Yoga was as much present here as in India. There are many other proofs which we haven't yet found but they are certainly there. It is necessary to go over to Pyandzh, Adzhinateppa, Pendzhikent and Afghanistan to find the full answers of above questions. But here our aim is not all that. We are simply concerned with making it clear that the existence of Yoga was there in our surroundings in the past as well but we were not aware of its presence so far.

Why was I born between the multi coloured high and Rocky Mountains in the north of Tajikistan, especially among backward, illiterate people and not in India or in any other advanced region? The most interesting thing is that, just not going to India, not having got acquainted with some Indian Yoga teachers and not having been taught by eminent yogis, I have become a master yogi, have left my prestigious specialist job of the professor of English in the University and have got totally engaged in Yoga only. Now nothing attracts me, but Yoga. I and my Yoga have become one, we are united forever.

Why I've been elected for this role? I simply wonder. I am ardently looking for its answer. And I do believe that it is there—just a little farther from me which I must know. May be, I am already on my way home!

2

MY LIFE, A MYSTERY TO ME

My life is a mystery to me from the beginning till today. While reading this book you'll make your own conclusions, no doubt, but let me utter at the outset, every step of my life is an imprint of the **invisible on me.**

I don't know what to begin with first, but it is necessary to start with something which you find interesting and worth your attention. It is impossible to learn the Tojik variant of Indian Yoga without going through my AUTO-BIOGRAPHY. My biography definitely shows what Tojik-Indian Yoga is. Why was I born between the wild high multi coloured high mountainous in the rear border village among totally illiterate backward people but incidentally shifted to the deeper world of wisdom coming from the southern side!

Once when I was sitting at the first International Yoga Conference in the 10th all India Yoga Championship in Talcatora Stadium, New Delhi in 1991, in which one Yoga scientist and a well known Yoga expert told me that Yoga has come to India from North, I. e. from Tajikistan or Afghanistan. Thinking that he was joking, I smiled and didn't take it seriously. Now I understand it better and might say that he was right in a way as there are so many statues in different postures (asanas) found now in our country.

Since I'd come across Yoga, I have transformed myself. Slowly, slowly, step by step I've changed myself into a totally positive man—mild as well as the man fighting for better life, according to Yoga philosophy, of course. I have turned myself like Viktor Gugor, who said: "Alive fight, but alive are only those, whose hearts are dedicated for a high daydream".

Now I have left teaching English as my profession of assistant professor at the University (in 2004) and have nothing to do with any practical and scientific activities of my profession and past life. My doctorate dissertation though ready with a great discovery in linguistics (the comparatives of English, Russian and Tojic), the monographs of dissertation are published, and three textbooks of "English for everybody", "English for beginners" and English in 30 days are ready to be published, does not attract me. I read no other books, but Yogic literature. I've cancelled all my past life activity.

Do you think I've gone mad? On the contrary when I look around and see disorders, opposite way of life by non-yogis (and they are in majority!) I try to make them understand, the right way, the best way of life by publishing articles in papers and magazines, writing books in Tojic and Russian (now in English), speaking over radio, TV very many times, speaking among people in Yoga clubs, Yoga centres, Yoga institutes and Yoga academy in places like Rishikesh, Delhi, Bhopal, Puttaparthy, Bangalore in India and in Russia or wherever I go.

3

DUSHANBE FOR STUDY

in 1968 I moved to Dushanbe to increase knowledge further. While being a post graduate research worker at the Academy of Sciences, I worked at the same Academy of science post graduate course, as the teacher of English for graduate students.

In 1973 I had presented the thesis on the subject of "The typology of the word order in the simple sentences of English, Russian and Tojik languages" successfully and became the candidate of the philological sciences.

I became an assistant professor of English, Russian and Tojik. First I worked at the Academy of Sciences for 9 years, then at the State University.

Coming to Dushanbe for study at the Post Graduate Course, I have stayed here ever since as it has given me everything I wished in my life: high knowledge, nice family with five wonderful children, very nice weather, Yoga and happiness. I lived in a leased apartment (flat) with my family of four persons: 2 little children, my wife and me. I worked at the Academy of Sciences at the chair of foreign languages, teaching post graduate students while me studying as a post-graduate course student. It was difficult to work and study in a small house. But I could manage to do so and in March 1973 I became an assistant professor of philological sciences much ahead of my turn.

That day (March the 8th 1973): I breathed heavily, deeply and remembered:

> "I breathed a song into the air;
> it fell to Earth I knew not where.
> I looked around, into my sphere,
> it brought me hardship everywhere.
> No more hardship for my family,
> No more shortages in my life.
> No more tears for my poor wife,
> No more misfortune I sworn twice.

I was the happiest of all men. My doctorate dissertation was half ready, I should have continued it but there was also the question of having my own house as my family had already suffered for long.

At the Academy of sciences where I worked, I was in the queue of getting a flat, but they went on postponing it. Wishing not to wait any longer, I decided to build a house myself. I turned myself into a builder and on the border (outskirts) of the Dushanbe city; I built a big house in a short time. I was an architect myself of this project.

There were so many tears, sorrows, but everything had now passed. After that there came the difficulty of finding the work for me in Dushanbe educational establishments.

While working as an assistant professor of English at the National University, I was not satisfied with teaching English at our schools and universities of Tajikistan. I wrote many articles in papers how to correct the situation, criticized the Minister of Education. Everywhere at the high educational establishments, they then refused me any work. I had to feed my big family anyhow. For a year I worked at the evening school where my children studied. One year I worked as an administrative rector of chancellery of the Institute of Art.

But the salary was not enough to feed my family. What to do? There came an idea to find work outside. I looked through advertising newspaper of "Uchitelskaya Gazeta" (Teachers' newspaper) and found the vacancy of the professor of English in Pavlodar (in the north of

Kazakhstan). Not delaying any further, I sent my required documents. In 27 days there came the answer to come and begin working.

It was the main reason of my going to Pavlodar. At that time I was sad and not satisfied for being there, but after coming across Yoga teachings, I was glad. This made me to come to the conclusion that all the hardships of life for me were well planned by the GOD HIMSELF!

I am very happy that I learnt Yoga somehow. May be otherwise, I had not known Yoga at all. I should have been just another person now that way, original, a bucket of diseases, and not a yogi!

Thank you, my GOD. You are really omniscient, omnipresent and omnipotent!

Now I know that you had sent me to Pavlodar to give me the key of yoga treasure house. Thank you so much again, my Lord!

Now I know that every step of me is under your observation. Now I know how you teach me, what to do, where to go, etc.

My dear readers! Do you understand now, why am I writing this book? I am under the security and protection of the All Mighty God Himself. He is same for everyone, but everyone does not know who he is and how best he is being taken care of by the Supreme! Until you don't find yourself, you won't find GOD either. This is the greatest secret of all secrets! For this purpose you must become a truthful, disciplined, obedient, positive, helpful, nice and thorough gentle man. God loves all positive people much greater.

Since 1985, I have combined Yoga with it (Karmyoga) till 2004. Slowly and slowly I felt myself to be a stranger at work, and didn't do my work rather seriously. I began to work formally to get money. But I didn't like it. I should have to procure doctoral thesis. It was ready for that. I had written some books for this. There appeared some difficulties while doing that. At last I understood that God doesn't want me be a doctor of sciences as I'll be fully busy with the academic life and won't pay much attention to Yoga. Then I came to the conclusion that I had to leave my work totally and be busy only with YOGA. It was a right decision as I find it now.

In 2004 I left my job at the University with 30 dollars as my pension per month . . . .

Till now, afterwards, I am busy only doing Yoga trainings with citizens of Dushanbe, writing articles on papers, writing books—all about Yoga and Indian way of life, the best way of living! I am all in all for Yoga only. Nothing interests me more than Yoga.

—Was my meeting with Mishra, P. D. just incidental?

—No, it was well planned by my destiny and the God!

Among 20 cooperative workers from India, only Mishra was a Yoga specialist. And he inviting me to India immediately and not letting me spend a penny during my two months stay there!

—Who can do this?

—Only a true yogi just by God's design!

It was God's plan to send one Yoga specialist for me to help! He is helping me up till now, and whatever I wish, He offers me happily.

In 1986 God's invisible presence prompted me to make it known that the USSR will be ruined and disintegrated. Not anticipating much about it, I wrote an open letter to Moscow newspaper "Izvestiya" to make my prediction public in the entire Soviet Union. I sent it on 10th September1986. On October the 3rd, 1986, under No. 104-205915, there came an answer:

"We don't send letters to the Central Committee of the USSR. You may send it there yourself".—Y. Gavrilov.

I was not much surprised that they had not believed in my prediction. I did not feel dejected, however, and looked for other via media to warn the society and the head of the Government. I particularly undertook the

10

onerous task of at least keeping alert my friends in Tajikistan so that they can avoid suffering during the changeover. That is why; I personally met and talked with our leaders of the state at that time particularly Rahmon Nabiev and Goibnazar Pallaev. They first agreed with me and promised to take some measures, but virtually did not.

Three times I had tried to meet our present President Emomali Rahmon, having sent him my own program and offers. Quite often I emerged on television and radio, warning people about the imminent. Widely I used foreign press, concretely analyzing unhealthy situation in the society and indicating the way out from the crisis. I also sent one letter to the UN. I sent it from India, when I was there in 1992.

I have published about 200 articles in English, Russian, Tojik, Byelorussian and Indian languages about human health happiness and well being. I took active participation in four international conferences of Yoga in Moscow, Dushanbe and India. I was a councilman to the Association of the USSR Yoga. I have been conferred and honoured with several degrees and diplomas in the Yoga conferences of the international order. I delivered lot many lectures in public in Moscow, Minsk, Tashkent, Tajikistan and India. I have organized myself one International Conference of the Yoga (2003) under the aegis of the embassy of India Yogendra Kumar in Embassy of the India in Tajikistan.

I am herewith reproducing my letter written to M. S. Gorbachov.

"OPEN LETTER TO:

The SECRETARY GENERAL
Central Committee of the Communist Party of the USSR
(M. S. GORBACHOV)

Dear Mikhail Sergeevich!

Finally, the time has come to live by the Lenin way. I see you are animated by Lenin once again. That is why, not being afraid, I herein write to you straight!

As SECRETARY GENERAL, I like you very much. I attentively follow your appearances and the policy.

What has forced me to write to you now? Your last appearance on television on All-union counsel managing pulpit of the public sciences under the slogan—"Learn on new to think and act". It was all inspiring. This was and it is my day dream as well.

I work in a high school since 1958. I cannot just accept the present status of imparting knowledge in our "developed socialism" of modern stage.

I say: "now what has happened in 5 years, no USSR will be there again, never will it be one so"!!!

"Emphasizing "fortification relationship of the theory with practice" You confirm that "This is the key to realignment . . .". Yes, you are absolutely true, but under one condition. It is necessary to change the structured base through physical improvement, in fascinating forced order.

We have become the slaves of our belly. Fat shrouds all our body, even our brain, exhausting us by poison. Forgive me for frankness, but such brain is not capable to think correctly. It is constantly occupied by the condition of its own defect, illness. It has no time for new thinking;

After all, "In a sound (healthy) body only there is a sound mind and the spirit".

TRULY YOURS

dedicated to the deal of the society as its servant,

Abduvahob Muhamadovich Sobirov, Assistant professor of the chair of the foreign languages of the Tojik Pedagogical Institute of the Russian language and Literature.

Dushanbe, September 10, 1986.
734036, 265, district 40 years of October, Dushanbe, Tojik SSR.

Sobirov, A. M.
I Z V E S T I Y A—October 3, 1986r. No. 104-205915

4

PAVLODAR FOR WORK

One day I was looking and reading the paper "Uchitelskaya Gazeta" ("Teacher's Paper") for the whole USSR Republics' readers. There were the advertisements of the vacant work at different republics' institutes and universities. I chose the Pavlodar Pedagogical Institute of English Department of Kazakh Republic as an assistant professor on competitive base. I sent there the documents

In less than a month, there came an invitation for me to come quickly and start working. I left my family in Dushanbe and went there to work. There they received me hospitably, provided a room in the hostel for teachers. The chair of the English Faculty was short of a qualified teacher. I quickly conquered the faith of the authorities among other competitors. It was 1983.

At that time I was a sick person: often having headaches, heart problems, throat diseases, backaches and leg problem, etc. For the sake of getting rid of them, I used to run 3 km in a day in the morning and did many other exercises, but it didn't help me much.

After a year of work here, I came across a yogi by chance in 1984. We were visited by a professor of English from Moscow called Sergay Migintessov who was in India with his father working in the Embassy of the USSR. Sergay had learnt Yoga well there. He had a certificate of the Yoga teacher as well.

There was one day a knock at my door of the hostel where I lived. I opened the door quickly.

—Are you Abduvahob Muhammadovich Sobirov?

The Russian gentle man whom came from Moscow like me as a professor of English was standing in front of me. He had his room next to me.

—Yes, you are not mistaken.

I answered at once.

—Are you a yogi?

He asked me for certain.

—What?!

I was astonished.—A "yogi", what is it?

—You see, it is an Indian way of living. It is performed by Indians, twisting their bodies in different postures, if you happened to see in some films!

—Ah! That monkey like fools, you mean?—

Suddenly it came out from my mouth.

—Oh, no! They are not fools as you imagine. They are absolutely very nice people, just living differently.

—Come in, please. Don't stay at the door.

I invited him to come in and sit, but he refused, saying he is in hurry.

—I shall come later and we'll continue our talk, said he and went away.

He came an hour later and we continued our talk.

—You are Sergey if I'm not mistaken, aren't you?

—Yes, I am.

—I'm Abduvahob, as you know. Now please tell me, who told you that I'm a "yogi"?

—The teachers of the English Department say that there's one more yogi at the Faculty, meaning you. They told that in the sauna you sit in "Padmasana" posture.

—What is "Padmasana"? I hear it for the first time.

—It is like this, said he and showed it by sitting on the floor.

—Ah! I sit there a little different, like this, said I and showed it also sitting on the floor.

—It is our "Chorzonoo". We always sit on the floor like this for taking our food, but this is more difficult as you show.

I tried like he showed, but couldn't.

—You sit in "Sukhasana".

—Now tell me Sergey, what is it that you call Yoga?

—Firstly, it is not mine, it is India's. I learnt how they perform the Yoga postures. Do you know that there are 8 millions & 400 asanas?

—Where could I know them from? What are they for?

—They are for curing diseases, increasing the life energy and as well concerning some other deep spiritual matters.

—Can you show me any Yoga secrets?

I began to be interested in Yoga.

16

He stretched his right hand index finger, tightened it and asked me to touch it. I did so, and momentarily took away my hand. His finger was as hot as iron taken from the fire.

—How did you make it like that?

I asked astonishingly.

—It's Yoga meditation.

—What is it?

—It is to think properly and concentrate your mind on a point or subject. Here I have concentrated and sent much blood to my index finger, that's all. You may exercise and learn also, said he seriously.

—Sergey, I see you are again in a hurry. Tomorrow is Sunday; won't you come to me to have dinner? I'm a nice cook; I'll prepare our wonderful "Pilaf" food. You'll like it.

—All right. I'll come, but for a short time. Now I have a meeting with some of our teachers on the matter of Yoga. See you tomorrow. Good bye.

After he left my room I was thinking much about "Yoga". I slept little that night; I wanted to know all about "Yoga". That Sunday morning I got up early and went to the grocery shop for shopping. I bought a kilogram of nice fatty sheep meat, 1 kg. Rice, 1 kg. Carrot, 1 kg. onion, butter, some fruits, hot drinks also, etc.,—all necessary items for a nice and rich dinner for two persons. Exactly at one o'clock there was a knock at my room's door. Sergey hurriedly entered, not waiting for me to open the door and sat at the dinner table. On seeing the table he was shocked and said:

—Oh, Abduvahob! Will there come some other quests? The table is covered for not a couple of people, but a dozen!

—No, none others will come, we are alone, will have as much as we can. What will you have for hot drink, "Russian vodka" (I think there were wine and Champaign too)?—On the big plate there was a nice "Pilaf" with meat inside the rice small cut. He thought for some time not knowing what to say. At last he uttered softly and kindly:

—Abduvahob, my dear friend, if you allow me to say so! Don't get offended on me if I shall have nothing of these on the table, but some fruit and tea with sugar with your permission.

—Why will you not have such a nice Pilaf and some drink? With Pilaf, drinking is pleasant, you see.

—Oh, my dear! Yogis won't have hot drinks and meat products at all.

—They are fools then. How to live without these products?—I was astonished and didn't understand what he meant.

—Abduvahob, have yourself what you wish here. Let's start,—and he put his hands with palms together on his chest, said something with his lips (now I know what prayer he said before meals), then had tea with bread, sugar, some fruit. I had my tasty Pilaf a little, drinking a glass of "Russian vodka".

—Dear friend,—he said again softly,—I'll give you a book for some time, you read it, then we shall talk again, O. K.?

—All right, you do that quickly.

—Wait a minute.—He went out and in 5 minutes brought a thick book by Dhirendra Brahmachary—"Yoga science".

—Read it attentively, after that you'll tell me your opinion, all right? Keep the book locked, don't show it to anyone else.

—All right, Sergey. Don't worry.

I read the book turning the pages slowly and slowly. It attracted my attention from the very start i.e. from the foreword which was written by Indira Gandhi, the Prime Minister of India. She said that the author of the book was her Guru, the Guru of her children as well as the Guru of her father, the former Prime Minister of India late Shri Jawahar Lal. She said that the book is wonderful in meaning, it's written for wide ranging readers of the world and it's easy for understanding. "It is very important and useful for curing the diseases", she stated. I couldn't stop reading it that night till the morning.

That day I didn't prepare for my lessons as they were formally completed. After the lessons were over, I quickly went to the dining-room, had lunch (we say "dinner") hurriedly (I had no breakfast, having no spare time) and went to the hostel, took the book, and continued reading further. Up to the late evening I finished it and lying down on my bed began thinking. The very first reaction of mine was: "What a fool I was while telling 'they are monkeys and fools' to Sergey. It's really a wonderful book of a wonderful Yoga philosophy and practical way of life. I must find this book for myself . . ."

Early in the morning, I knocked Sergey's door. He opened it chewing something in his mouth (he was having breakfast). I begged pardon for my ill behaviour during our first meeting and not returning him the book I asked him to leave it for some more days. He said that it was impossible as the other teachers were in turn going to read that book further.

—Is it possible to find and buy from somewhere the book?—I asked him anxiously.

—It's impossible you see. It was published secretly by the order of some people in Russia. There are one or two in Moscow, in Leningrad and some other cities of the USSR. Here only I have it. It's not sold anywhere.

—Oh! What's a pity! I must have it anyhow. I urgently ask you to leave the book for a few more days. Let others wait a little, dear Sergey? I beg your pardon.

—O. K., only two or three days, Abduvahob. You are welcome, have a breakfast with me.

—Thank you, I have fried eggs for my breakfast. Little time is left to go to the Institute. I do not have time to prepare to the lessons, you see. The book has engaged me so much. Good bye, dear Sergey.

That day I had one lesson. Being not prepared to the subject, I asked the students to read the book about the history of London while I was reading the Yoga book again. At the end of the lesson we discussed a little what they had read and hurriedly I went home.

Again hurriedly, I had my dinner out of the food left in the evening, took a thick notebook and started to make a copy of the book. At that time there was no copying machines and I had nothing to do, but copy it this way only. Of course I made a copy of the summary of the book. It took me a week. Asanas also I drew on the copying paper. I gave the book back and started to learn the Yoga asanas and Pranayam for my diseases. Firstly, my headache stopped to disturb me and then my backache disappeared. It made me brave. I stopped my sports exercises and did only Yoga practices seriously. My diseases left my body one after one. I became much stronger than before. Seeing me that I was so much interested in Yoga, Sergey gave me a photo film, saying there is another Yoga book photographed in it that I might reproduce on photo papers and use it also. Now I had two Yoga books. They made me understand Yoga better.

I also asked my students whether they knew anything about Yoga, if they had seen somewhere something about Yoga and collected clippings of papers and magazines about Yoga anytime, anywhere but there was no positive response.

Thus Pavlodar played a great role in my lifespan. It widened my knowledge. Virtually, it opened my inner world, the hidden world of my past life. Now I am sure that in the past life I definitely lived in India, in Bhopal region perhaps, and was the follower of Buddha. Pavlodar opened a new page in the book of my life span. In Pavlodar I met yogi Sergay only 3 times: firstly, when he knocked at my door for asking whether I was a yogi, secondly, when he had come to me for having a dinner, and thirdly, when he gave me a photo film and said "Good bye" before my departure from Pavlodar to Dushanbe. That's all. He didn't teach me yoga as it is. Everything I achieved is just by practicing, reading books, newspaper clippings etc.

A real Yoga has thus sprout out from me as it is . . . . I've written about 10 books on yoga in Tojik and Russian. Now I've written this book in English with the help of P. D. Mishra with whom we have cooperated very much on Yoga path in Tajikistan and in India. I and Mishra have published many articles in papers of Tokikiston and India (some of them we have reproduced in this book). In my country I've published about 150 articles in Tojik and in Russian on yoga way of life. For Yoga to be popularised in my country, I've left my profession of 'professor of English' at the University in 2004. Now I'm busy only with Yoga practices and principles among the citizens of my country. It'll continue till the end of my life. Now I sleep just for 3 hours at night. After I get up at 3-4 o'clock in the morning, I'm busy with Yoga—Hath and Raja. I care for no other work or book, but Yoga. I think, do, write, speak on Yoga anyhow, anywhere, everywhere and wherever I am among people. Everybody in my city, country and abroad, knows and wishes me to teach and discuss Yoga only.

5

BACK TO DUSHANBE

After some days of my arrival to Dushanbe my wife Habiba, who had suffered very much for my being away, told me that in a week my elder daughter Husniya would have an operation of her throat for the sore throat. And our elder son Alisher would have a serious operation of his testicles. One of them fell 7 centimetres down. In the hospital he has been put in a queue, his turn would come in May of 1986. All your children are ill with one or the other disease and they are week in study at school as well for want of proper care.

—My dear Habiba! There will be no more doctors and operations, no tablets to be taken for diseases, no more problems, but me with my yogasanas and strict discipline, you see. I have learned the interesting method of curing any disease.

—"Yugsans"? What is it? You are a teacher of English, what it concerns with medicine? You'd better leave that "Yugsans" of yours. If something wrong would happen with them? What shall we do then? My dear husband, you better concern yourself with your English and do your doctorate dissertation.

She was absolutely ignorant of my telling such a thing. I explained to her in a simple way what "Yoga" means. She knew of my diseases and had by now understood that my health had remarkably improved.

—Habiba! My dear wife, don't worry any more about your children's diseases. They will be cured by me, you'll see yourself. I'm not telling a lie. I'm sure what is what now. I've turned myself to be a doctor, a nice one and certainly not like many others. I'm a doctor without tablets and chemicals, injections, operations, etc.

I talked with my children seriously also and asked them to get up at 6 o'clock in the morning. They were five: two daughters and three sons. Every day we did pranayama and special yogasanas together. Not before long, they became enough strong. I taught the lion posture to my daughter Husniya for her sore throat. In 10 days she became quite well and didn't complain about her throat any longer. When my wife took her to the doctors, they were astonished on seeing no problem with her throat. My wife began to believe me and made no obstacle in my Yoga methods afterwards.

I took with my elder son Alisher who expected a serious operation. There were 6 months left, he was under doctor's control, and he took medicine. For him I used maximum asanas and pranayama with special performance of Paschimottanasana and Bhujangasana. The doctor examining him after six months was amazed on finding no problem in my son's body. He was also much stronger than before.

Thus I came to a conclusion that I might do away with medicines altogether and can bring revolution. I looked for extension of my experience. There were some of my relatives who were suffering from heart diseases all the time and very often they lay in the hospitals for curing. Once I called them to my house to be my quests for a serious discussion on the problem of their diseases. It was Sunday, they came, all three of them: Colonel Rustam Abdulloev, assistant professor of Tajikistan history Muhammadjon Rahmadjonov, assistant professor of pedagogic Naimjon Sanginov. I told them that they wouldn't get rid of their diseases by medical cure. They would be worse and worse . . . There is a Yoga method which I learned in Pavlodar of Kazac Republick by chance, made myself and my children absolutely healthy. I proved it calling my wife for bearing the witness. At last I told that they might be cured without any tablets very soon under my management. They consented. I asked them to come every Sunday at 7 o'clock having no breakfast. They'd have it after yoga training in an hour in my house.

Thus, we gathered on the veranda of my house for about six months once a week. They became better and better. They all had heart problems and they were not allowed to lift anything heavy. After five month I learned that Rustam had lifted a sack of potatoes to his compartment on the third floor, the others were busy with hard physical work. They had forgotten about their heart problems.

It was Rustam Abdullocv who had twice micro heart problem but was always faithful to jump, raise some heavy things, and move abruptly, etc. after two months of Yoga exercises he lifted a sack of potatoes to the third floor of his flat. The second was Naimjon Sanginov by name, formerly my student in Leninabad. After he left English and passed to the Pedagogic subject and worked at the Ministry of the public education. After 2 months of Yoga exercises with me he began to build a house, doing hard physical work. I have seen him by my own eyes as his house is just 50 meters away my house.

Here was the third, Muhammadjon Rahmadjonov, assistant professor of Tajikistan History. While writing his doctorate dissertation in his dacha around Dushanbe he was accidentally shot down and killed by a Government officer who was looking for rebel fighter.

At last there came an idea. I decided to spread my experience among the people of my country. I wrote an article for the Russian paper "Communist of Tojkistan" and named it "The golden key of Health". There came cheers of surprise by phone. Then I wrote the second and the third article in series explaining the importance of Yoga for everybody, for every disease. There came some people and asked me to work with them.

I was highly glad. I began to think what to do further. I meditated in my garden on the cot for a long time. We looked for a hall. 10 interested persons came there. Nobody of them knew what Yoga is. I always explained it by simple words. Day by day they felt themselves better. I drew a big plan of expansion of Yoga in the country and went to the second secretary of the Central Region of Dushanbe City asking her for opening a Yoga cooperative, but she didn't consent and told me to approach the Ministry of Health.

When I went to the Minister of Health Gulnora Kamilovna for help of using Yoga curing method among the population under the guidance of the Ministry of Health she said proudly:

—Who are you and what is it "Yoga"? You tell me about it in detail?

—I am professor of English at the University, but Yoga is a curing method of diseases which I learned and have got some experience. It is my hobby now. There are 10 patients who are being cured by me. Here are some articles written by me in these papers about Yoga. I stretched them to her.

—There it is written and demonstrated what Yoga is.

She took the papers, overturned them hurriedly, then returned them to me back and seriously addressed me:

—Firstly, you are not a medical worker; you have nothing to do with medicine. Go and teach your English at the University. Secondly, you say Yoga is an exercise. Then go to the sports Committee, sports clubs. May be they'll help you. You have no medical certificate either.

—Anyhow if you allow me to open a Yoga cooperative I'll prove myself to make it very useful, I urged and said emphatically.

—No, it's impossible, I've no time, and we have a meeting of doctors now . . . .

I got angry that she didn't understand me. Looking at her I made a conclusion that she was absolutely illiterate in the matter of Yoga. She was very fat and she scarcely fitted in her armchair. I came to the idea that she was totally ill. She was so fatty that she could hardly breathe while talking with me. I stood up unsatisfied and left her study closing her door powerfully.

Going home I was thinking what to do next. I didn't have any wish to leave Yoga activity. I decided to write a critical story in the paper about our talk with the Minister of Health Gulnora Kamilovna. That day till late at night I wrote and finished the article and in the morning I took it to the editor of the paper "Kommunist Tajikistan". The editor read it attentively and surprisingly told me that it's a bomb shell for the Ministry of Health.

—It's a good critique, my dear—said the editor. He was a Russian man recently nominated from Moscow here. He thought a little, turned to me and in all certainty said:—If you let me do, we shall moderate it a little and I'll write my opinion at the end.

—I agree,—said I.—I must open a cooperative of health in Dushanbe, because it's an easy method of curing patients without tablets and chemicals.

—I know Yoga a little. You are right, I shall help you, believe me.

He was cultured, literate in Yoga, honest and a truthful man. I liked him. I was satisfied on our talk.

—It'll be published very soon. Then we shall see.

I was very glad and happily went home. In three days my article was published. It brought a resonance among people. There were many calls and questions for me. I felt myself a revolutionary man. Such a reality was brought out in words in our country for the first time. Everybody was shocked on my brave appearance in public with such a serious problem of life. By this time I had found some more books on Yoga and my knowledge was increased. I was sure what I had said.

But having no certificate for Yoga was a problem. At these moments there appeared a Russian man who was in India for some time, went to the Yoga club sometimes and had a certificate of a Yoga instructor.

We decided with him to work together for opening a Yoga cooperative in Dushanbe. After my article was published the second secretary of the Central Region with whom we had met and but had refused me to open the Yoga cooperative, called me saying:

—Why have you criticized me?—There I had mentioned her as after refusing, she had sent me to the Ministry of Medicine.

—I only wished you to bring me the Minister's consent.

—Excuse me; the truth is always the truth.

—All right. I see you won't let the matter remain subsided. Prepare documents for setting up a Yoga cooperative in some policlinics of the city, where you wish. Bring them quickly, please.

This time she was polite enough. I believed that she had a talk with the Minister of Health and had decided to get rid of me; otherwise I'd be criticizing them again.

From there straight I went to our policlinics No. 8, knocked at the door of the head doctor Esan Tadjibaev and entered. He invited me politely to have a seat. We were not acquainted before. I introduced myself and told the aim that had brought me to him.

—You say "Yoga", what it is; I don't know it at all. Will you bring me something to read for making clear what it is?

—Why not, I'll bring you the books to read. You know I may cure the patients without tablets by a special Yoga method. It'll be of much help for you also.

—All right then.

—I'll bring them now. said I and quickly went home. I brought two books and my published articles in papers. He took them and said:

—Come in three days, please.

When I went after three days he gave his consent without any objection. He was kind and hospitable. I guess that the higher authorities had directed him to give his consent without any objection. Esan Tadjibaev said:

—You may begin your work in our physical culture hall at any time comfortable to you. You may write and hang the timetable on the door. Let anybody whosoever wishes, come there. Abduvahob, mind one thing:

our therapeutic head doctor would come to the Yoga training classes and control the patient's health.

—All right, Esan Tadjibaevich, you are very kind. Never mind, everything will be all right.

Thus, I won the battle on empty space, having no certificate of medical worker and Yoga. Now I had an official document for expansion of Yoga in Tajikistan. I knew that somebody from outside helped me and forced me to do this. It was the outer space command for this part of the world. They had chosen me since my birth in Bobodarkhan village, put in my mind the special program of my life through the path of which I had to discover the lost goal of past life. Now I have more than ten documents (certificates) of the highly qualified Yoga master from different parts of the world: Dushanbe, Moscow, Minsk and, India. I have many invitations from Africa, Germany, Polish, Moscow, and Minsk for the organization of my Yoga variant in their countries.

I was in India for ten times and have 10 diplomas of excellence from highly qualified Yoga masters. The first was given by P. D. Mishra in Dushanbe in 1989. Now I feel myself (in 2013) absolutely qualified who has nothing to do with anything else, but Yoga till the end of my life.

Thus I worked at the policlinics No. 8 of Dushanbe for about a year with patients who came from outside while teaching the doctors there as well. I had two groups there. Little by little they understood the importance of Yoga training for curing the diseases. I wrote article after article about my experience and the use of Yoga in papers and magazines, spoke over TV & radio many times. Everybody in Tajikistan learned what Yoga is and where it had come from.

When I analyze it where has it come from, I understand that from nowhere indeed as it was there and it is there and it'll be there until I'm there. I was born in the wild place of the North of Tajikistan for the purpose of proving me to be a messenger of Yoga in Tajikistan, firstly going nowhere to study it. Till now nobody taught me to do this or that. I read only the books and came to the conclusion that I can sincerely put my knowledge into practice. Now I invent yogasanas myself, I need not consult any book I read, I'm in no need of any outside world any more. I live in the Yoga world of my creation!

From the first few days of my early awakening nothing indeed was wrong in my steps taken. Anything difficult or wrong in my life was turned into right for me and only to undergo experiences of hard life for being careful in future. I remember how willingly sometimes I took many obvious wrong steps believing that they'll bring happiness in my life. For example, I tried to do business. Many times I tried to do it in India; even I took along a group of businessmen and tolerated total failure. Then urgently I wished to be a doctor. At last, when everything was ready for the presentation of the thesis, there was the outside command that there's no use for me of doing anything of this sort in my life. Now I'm busy only with Yoga activity among the citizens of Dushanbe and Tojkistan.

It's interesting to mention that any time I came to India, whenever I went to the Yoga clubs, Yoga centres, institutes in Bhopal and Delhi, the Yoga Academy in Rishikesh, they have asked me to teach their students my Yoga methods for sure. As a result they liked it and praised my teaching everywhere. After some days of my teaching, they gave me the certificate of excellence calling me a highly qualified Yoga master.

6

P. D. MISHRA PLAYS MAIN ROLE IN MY YOGA LIFE

In 1989 there appeared a cooperative delegation of 20 persons in Dushanbe from India. I was just wondering that there must be some Yoga master in it with whom I might discuss some of my misunderstandings in Yoga.

One day I incidentally entered the central hospital to see my sick friend. Just at that moment the doctors were looking for someone who knew English for interpreting an Indian patient saying something whom they had brought for cure. On seeing me the doctor was glad (as she knew me to be the English specialist) and asked to see an Indian patient and learn what the problem was with him. I learned that something was wrong with his nose—the haemorrhoid. Learning that he was not a yogi I explained him to get cured by Yoga method better and told how to go for it. As a result of my consultation he became alright.

Then I asked him whether there was any one who knew Yoga in his delegation. He thought a little and said:

—I don't exactly know because we are from different cities of India, but may be the head of our delegation is one as I saw him once meditating. Give me your address, please, I shall ask him and send him to you, if he wishes.

—Be that kind to do so. I need some Yoga expert very much.

Just in a day, unexpectedly there came to my Yoga centre the head of the Indian delegation, P. D. Mishra. He was surprised seeing Yoga activities going on in Dushanbe. Later on he helped me much by his advises, speeches about Yoga among my disciples and citizens, answering their questions. I took him along with other members of his delegation to my house many times. We indeed became good friends.

P. D. Mishra was one and the first Indian expert on Yoga who returning to India from Dushanbe in 1989 invited me to visit India which he had promised me.

By that time, I had been to Egypt and some other countries of the world, but India I liked most from the very first glance. It was right that Mark Twain said: "Who has seen India once, he will never wish to visit any other country in the world". It was Mishra who took me here and there to the places of interest all over India, not letting me pay a penny anywhere. He sponsored my visit every time in India. Thus he played a wonderful and vital role in my Yoga path.

I firmly believe that I lived here in India (Bhopal) in my past life. I found here many dearest friends who in my past life were surely my very dear relatives.

At the Bhopal State Yoga Institute we exchanged opinions, cooperated and worked together in harmony for evolving it as a common way. Girish Khare was the director of the Yoga Institute and he conferred on me a diploma of a master of Yoga in 1991. It has become my first official document ever since on Yoga in my country, though while in Dushanbe Mishra had given me a letter of appreciation about my positive contribution in the field there.

During my first visit to India I became a participant of the 10th national all India Yoga championship which took place in Talcatora Stadium in Delhi. There I met many Yoga teachers, masters, scientists, gurus who opened my eyes wide on Yoga. Mehta took me there; he also accompanied me to Dahisar Village to meet Swami Shivom Tirth who became my guru also. Since then his photo is hanging on the wall of my bedroom with a nice white and long beard. Mehta accompanied me to Rishikesh also. This is a wonderful place in the world I think. I loved this place very much, that is why I visited it thrice afterwards.

P. D. Mishra took me to Satya Sai Baba in Puttaparthy whom I knew nothing about except some of his sayings which Mishra was often referring to from his writings and speeches. On seeing him in Prashanty Nilayam during darshan hours I didn't believe in his miracles, especially when he was producing vibhuti. I thought it was some trick. In a week we returned back to Bhopal. In the train I got ill seriously. My body was shivering with strong fever.

During this first visit to India I gathered much literature about Yoga and Sai Baba which made me rich in knowledge. What I learned out of this literature and what I saw by my eyes in India, I started to write articles for papers and magazines in my country. I wrote a lot about Sai Baba as I began to believe in Him. I wrote about His life and activities, miracles, vibhuti etc.—about 30 articles in various papers.

After I came back from India, my activity on Yoga path increased. I went to Tojik radio and television. My Yoga trainings were regularly shown by TV. Tojikistonians liked and loved my Yoga classes. Many people came to Yoga centres. In Dushanbe itself I had 10 Yoga centres. In the centre of all regions of Tojik Republic these centres were working. The reality is also this that nobody has financed us or sponsored till now. I do it myself, on my own initiative, gathering some donations on charity from disciples. I have never stopped Yoga trainings with the people who come to my Yoga centre three days a week for one hour.

Thus, I became little interested in my job—teaching English language at the University. Now I am occupied only in Yoga, writing articles, books, training citizens in curing (Yoga therapy), etc. Now everybody in the Republic of Tajikistan knows me and respects me. I don't slow down my activity in this field any way. We do not have our own building for yoga purposes. Still I feel that some power makes me go ahead and do my best in Yoga and to never stop there.

By Mark Twain's mind, I didn't stop going to India. I visited it again and again. It is my jubilee, i.e. the 10th visit to India (2013).

I visited Sai Baba in Puttaparthy 4 times; lastly I had been living there for 40 days. In the morning of the last day, before my departure, Baba called me for the interview which continued for one hour. At the end, He presented me a cosmic ring with three brilliant jewels which I wear till now. Once I lost one jewel but soon found it again. Twice I lost the ring itself, but found it back in a day. I was so much upset then. I could understand that Baba was playing with me a trick and checking my patience, my belief in Him. Here is the ring:

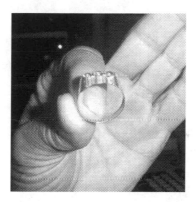

PART TWO

Keys, Instructions and Reclamations

1

EVERYONE CAN DO IT

If you strictly follow my recommendations, without any doubt, observe all rules and laws of Yoga, change your former, wrong way of life, sincerely believe in me and live as explained here, you will definitely achieve all your goals, i. e. All that mankind has been looking for from the very start of life.

Following are the objectives you generally set for your life:

1. To be always happy and healthy.
2. To be well preserved for life long activity.
3. To not to get old and be young till the end of life.
4. To become just immortal.

OPTIMISM OVERCOMES PESSIMISM, AND WISDOM OVERCOMES EVIL.

YOUR BELIEF (FAITH) IS THE GUARANTEE OF YOUR SUCCESS!

There is no other truth truer than this one!

"If this be error and upon me proved, I never writ, not any man ever loved"—Shakespeare.

"Alive are fighting, and alive are only those whose hearts are devoted to the elevated goal"—V. Gyugo.

TRUTH IS ONE AND IT MAY BE ACHIEVED BY THOSE WHO ARE TRUE BELIEVERS.

THE ASHTANGA YOGA ASSURES HUMAN BEING'S HAPPINESS AS ABOVE AND PROVIDES TRUTHFUL LONGEVITY.

I wish you the biggest success!!!

2

INSTRUCTIONS

Yogic Rules of behaviour for everyday life

1. **The basic reason of any disease** is insufficient amount of oxygen in the blood, insufficient physical exercises, wrong diet, overeating, alcohol, tobacco (chewing, smoking), salt, sugar (refined) and most of all slaughtered and toxin food products, such as meat, chemicals, drugs, etc.

2. You should change your way of life into simple, cheaper and straight for being always healthy, young, by following the golden yogic way of life.

3. Go to bed by 10-11 o'clock and sleep not for more than 6 hours.

4. Sleep on plane and hard place (bed), better on the floor without chink between the wood boards.

5. Do Yoga exercises on empty stomach in the morning, or before meal (dinner) in the evening.

6. You must be always hygienic, clean both from outside and inside your body, i. e. wash yourself (your body) and take shower, bath (warm) in the morning, but before performing Yoga training. You may do it after 2 hours of Yoga training, but not earlier.

7. If you have no facility to take shower you may slightly wash your hands and face.

8. Observe nonviolence of any living creature both by words and deeds, and even by mind (thought). One must not wish anyone anything wrong.

9. Be always truthful, sincere, disciplined and modest.
10. Do not take any body's possession without permission; never steal away anything of others.
11. Do not collect big amount of money and material things for tomorrow, i. e. Do not provide much for a rainy day; don't think of tomorrow at all. "Tomorrow will take care of itself by itself. We have got enough misery for today". Thus was the testament of Christ, the God.
12. Here is one of the best commandments: "Oh God, give me peace, teach me to reconcile with that which I can't change; and let me differ in wisdom from one another".
13. Believe the Super Intelligence-Truth, Nature, Cosmos, Spiritualism; otherwise without such belief your life is a tragic farce.
14. One of the greatest spiritualists of India ever since Buddha's time, Mahatma Gandhi, wrote: "Without praying I should have been turned into a mad man long ago".
15. If you can't address God, then do it to someone of your high esteem, or simply address yourself, as the true reflection of God.
16. Regulate your sexual urges, calm down your mind, and abstain from involvement. It'll cure you from many diseases and disorders. Your willpower will become strong and you'll have healthy spirit.
17. Be satisfied with all that surrounds you—both good and bad. You must look at all things and at everybody from one point of view: as natural and the ultimate product of Nature.
18. Get rid of tight, synthetic, artificial clothes, narrow and high heeled shoes. They do not let you move naturally and obstruct harmonic energy flow in the body.
19. Do not bathe in the very cold and very hot water. The body will only suffer from it.
20. Sleep with open window on plane and hard place, floor or ground. You'll thus gain, not lose anything, because your sleep will be deep and doubly useful. Firstly, by resisting the hardness your body will automatically be strengthened; secondly, lying on plain bed the whole body, with all its parts inside, will be functioning correctly and supplying normal blood as well as the oxygen creating natural metabolism. Such kind of sleep of 3-4 hours is enough to feel oneself cheerful and healthy for the whole day.
21. Do Yoga regularly under any conditions and weather, and most of all, never be lazy in it.

22. Never do deep yogic breathing with your stomach filled up with food.

23. Learn Yoga breathing well. Always breathe right (pressing your uvula—little tongue—to the back part of your tongue in the throat) by nose. As it is impossible to eat by nose, it is the same—you are not allowed to breathe by mouth. When breathing is right the wings of the nose do not take part, they do not move. For this purpose lower down little tongue (uvula) on the root (base) of your tongue and slightly pressing it you'll hear hissing in the ear. Only this is the right breathing! You must learn always to breathe like this. At the beginning it'll be difficult and uneasy, but practicing regularly every day, you'll learn it in 3-5 days. Always remember that you are Microcosms and all laws of Macrocosms are put in your body in miniature. And your little tongue is a switch of Macro with Micro. Clear? If not, come up to me for more details in practice. All those who can't breathe like this live for a shorter span of life and always keep suffering from diseases.

24. Distinguish 4 types of yogic breathing: 1/ low, 2/ middle, 3/ up, 4/ deep, among which last one is the best one, as it is fuller, deeper. For supporting the body in normal healthy state one must take 60 deep breathing per day, dividing it into three times: 20 breathing (on empty stomach) in the morning, 20 breathing in the afternoon, 20 breathing in the evening.

25. Before going to bed one must do some deep breathing exercise (Pranayam).

26. Be patient; do not be in a hurry to achieve better results quickly. The main thing in Yoga is regularity and faith in success.

27. Before beginning the Yoga practice drink one glass hot boiled water (cleaned raw water). The same you must do before going to bed to sleep and also after getting up.

28. You must drink any liquid by swallowing, i. e. Sip slowly anything you drink, first keeping in the mouth for a while, and thus one should drink not less than 2 litters of water or any liquid per day.

29. One must not bolt, gulp down or gobble any liquid (quaff it). You must eat slowly chewing the food well. Do not be in a hurry, leisurely chew the food till it becomes juice or something like soft porridge moistening by saliva, and then swallow it slowly and slowly. It takes time of course, but you gain strength and longevity of life.

30. You must not drink tea or water (or any other liquid) during eating or after having had food till half an hour passes. You may drink them before 10 minutes of taking your food.
31. You must eat only when you feel a natural hunger and eat moderately, and certainly never overeating.
32. All those who do Yoga practice for the sake of achieving better health, may eat what they wish, if they can't do it any other way. However, they should gradually switch over to the prescribed order in a course of time.
33. Yoga disciple keeping strictly to the established order and discipline must confine to the strict vegetarianism.
34. Avoid fried food, too much boiled, white refined sugar, salt, onion and garlic.
35. Drink the fruit, berry, vegetable grass, greenery juices and vegetable clear soups.
36. Do not eat more than one food one time which contains starch.
37. Don't eat bread, potatoes, rice, and macaroni simultaneously.
38. In no case take many dishes at one time.
39. Monodite is the best way both for loosing flesh and feeling oneself healthy.
40. Better take vegetables, greens, fruit and berry raw, uncooked, i. e. fresh, and better to eat them, if you can, with skin, peel if you can't do so, then make out of them stuffing and chew mixing with saliva. With all you've got in your mouth, always mix it with saliva well. Don't drink while chewing and swallowing.
41. Do not eat meat and dishes made out of meat.
42. Remember: "One must only eat to live, but not live just to eat".
43. Once a day in a week fast for 24-26 hours. You may drink only clean water when you feel thirsty.
44. Remember the motto of yogis: "Clean air, clean food, clean yoga training and clean life forever!"
45. To get used to all this takes a month or a little more. It is as easy as that. It just depends on the true Yoga knowledge and the will power of a person.
46. Be an optimist and believe in success!
47. I am directing you to the kind, purple and wide road of Yoga longevity, my dear reader!
48. I am calling you to the golden tiny brooks of youth and immortality, oh my long suffering friend!

49. Remember the proverb and follow it at once: "NEVER PUT OFF TILL TOMORROW WHAT YOU CAN DO TODAY"!!!
50. DON'T LOOSE YOUR PRECIOUS CHANCE NOW AVAILABLE TO YOU SO CLOSE BY!!!
51. THE ADVICES GIVEN ABOVE ARE NOT FOR COMFORT AND PLEASURE, OR JUST FOR READING AND FORGETTING. THEY MUST BE FOLLOWED IN LIFE, APPLIED IN DAILY PRACTICE BY EACH AND EVERYONE WHO CHERISHES A DESIRE TO LIVE A HEALTHY HAPPY LIFE.

3

WHAT IS YOGA AND WHAT IT DOES TO A MAN?

Do you know that after 24 hours or more of your activity, your muscle tissues begin to deteriorate which takes you in to the trap of diseases silently?

There is only one way to prevent it or get rid of when caught after falling in the trap forever. That way is through Yoga and yogic training, carried out regularly at least 6 times a week. The minimum time required for a yogic activity to be really effective is 30 minutes early in the morning.

Yogic trainings are isotonic in nature, i. e. they involve the rhythmic movements of arms, legs and larger muscle groups of the body (bottom, back). These muscle groups are shortening and lengthening under performance of special asanas.

Thus, yogic activity puts your body as well as your heart under repeated and measured steady stress, i. e. it builds and increases its strength and stamina. Moreover, it increases one's overall fitness level.

Practically yogic training increases oxygen consumption which increases one's physical capacity, i. e. increases the conditions of the heart and lungs to perform their duties more effectively.

Yogic exercises performed well make one's skin and hair glow as life giving oxygen rushes all through capillaries under the skin all over the body, supplying them the nutrients and thereby improving the blood circulation which gives you a healthy appearance. They increase stamina, the body's endurance to work long and enduringly without fatigue.

Yogic training reduces free radicals in the blood vessels which otherwise create havoc in the body system accelerating and aggravating the ageing process; they make you look younger with fewer wrinkles.

Yogic training enlarges the blood vessels and strengthens the heart muscles increasing one's working capacity. Fatness goes away with the replacement of lean muscle with fatty tissues.

Yoga training makes one's body change slowly, giving it the proper shape and definition by preventing muscle shrinkage. They keep hormone levels high which is necessary for the skin. They also keep sexuality potentially healthy and high.

4

YOGA IS NO TOUCH THERAPY

Yoga has got a history of more than 5.000 years. Since its appearance long before it has now enough updating for its being truthfully most practical than any of the other later born sciences.

According to Yoga philosophy there is a universal energy which is called Prana. It is such an energy which is invisible and its life force surrounds the physical body of everyone. It surrounds the body like aura and penetrates deep into the body.

One must know that there are the energy body and the physical body in every living being. They are different but very closely related to each other. Prana is absorbed through the energy body and only then it is distributed throughout the entire physical body. This energy plays the role of safeguarding the body from bacteria, germs, chemicals which penetrate the energy body, where they are kept for about three months before they manifest in the physical body. Like the physical body where blood circulates in blood vessels, in energy body there are invisible channels called nadis through which Prana flows. This energy body has got 7 chakras which correspond to the vital organs in the physical body. When these chakras are balanced and harmonized only then the physical body will have the perfect health. Any imbalance in the chakras and nadis makes the person get ill.

Such diseases like tonsillitis, cough happen when bioplasmic throat is weak.

From whatever said above, we come to the conclusion that it is very easy to get rid of any disease in the physical body, if one scans the conditions of chakras and nadis which make the aura. After such diagnosis one may easily remove the disease by "cleansing" the energy and replenishing the body with fresh Prana which is vital energy. It is called "energizing". This kind of energy is usually taken from earth, water air, fire and ether—the five fundamental elements of nature.

While the aura is treated for bringing in balance, there is no physical contact with a patient in it. As such it is "no-touch Therapy" which is painless and does not need any drugs or equipment. The healing depends on how one is using the yogic practice, where and when, and whether complete or partial, regular or irregular, etc.

By this "yogic no-touch Therapy" all kinds of physical, emotional and mental diseases can be cured. For making this healing more effective it is very important for the patient to forget fear and despair. Also one must have faith and totally be open to receive the healing energy, otherwise the healing is restricted. Much success in healing depends on the efforts of the individuals and their teachers (instructors, gurus), under whose guidance they are being healed up.

Just be aware of the right knowledge and don't be in a hurry. Better to be slow, but steady and faithful.

5

CONTROLING DAILY DIET

What kind of food must one take per day usually? Do you know it? If you don't, then seriously take care of it for your wellness.

Since childhood we know a lot about organics and non-organics. For our food we must use only organic elements of food. Such kind of elements is contained in fruits, vegetables, juices, greenery, nuts, and cereals. If one wants to be quickly healthy enough he/she must eat only organic vegetarian food. For such purpose of quicker betterment from a lot many diseases and becoming beautiful, handsome, strong and all healthy person, I'll give you here A TEN DAY ELIMINATION DIET for everybody, especially for the obesity to be slim.

Mind that the biogenic-organic diet has got life penetrating powers. These kinds of foods (raw fruits, sprouts, vegetables, seeds, grains) help in proper elimination and detoxification of the body.

More than that, it helps to heal the dyeing cells and microorganisms of one's body. Organic raw (fresh) food products are always available with little or no chemicals in them, which contain all their nutritive value and taste.

Again, the way your daily food is being cooked: vegetables, grains (cereals), they do not give us any special benefit in the meaning of health. They only fill up the body with sustenance for much nonsense. It is just because one cannot help eating "the normal food" cooked at home "well" or outside more "deliciously". And nobody is sure that he/she is making daily mistake and it must not be the centre of the meal taken for the benefit of the body. As a rule, naturally it must be considered as a complimentary dish only.

We must not even talk about tinned, refined or concentrated as they are the containers of all the diseases in the body.

First day:

1. In the morning after washing and cleaning the body before Yoga training, drink 1 glass of boiled and warm or cleaned raw water.
2. At noon (12 o'clock): a) one glass of fresh orange juice. It may be changed into other juice you prefer. b) 1 glass of herbal tea (any).
3. In the afternoon (16 o'clock): 1 or 2 glasses of fresh vegetable juice. It may be changed, owing to the taste, by 1 bowl of fresh salad with curd.
4. In the evening (20 o'clock): a) the same as at noon: b) 1 small bowl of boiled rice with vegetable soup.
5. Go to bed having taken 1 glass of boiled or cleaned warm water (22 o'clock). It may be changed by herbal tea.

Second day:

1. It is the same as in the first day.
2. The same.
3. The same.
4. The same.
5. The same.

Third day:

1. It is the same as in the preceding days.
2. The same.
3. a) 1 glass of fresh juice (any); b) 2 boiled potatoes; c) a small bowl of curd.
4. The same as in the preceding days.
5. The same.

Fourth day:

1. The same as in the preceding days.
2. 2 glasses of any fresh fruit juice.
3. The same as in the preceding days.
4. The same.
5. The same.

Fifth day:

1. The same as in the preceding days.
2. The same.
3. The same.
4. 1 bowl of fresh vegetable salad.
5. The same as in the preceding days.

Sixth day:

1. The same as in the preceding days.
2. a) 1 glass of herbal tea. b) 2 glasses of fresh orange juice.
3. a) 1) 1 glass of fresh vegetable juice; b) 1 bowl of steamed vegetables; c) 1 bowl of sprouted salad.
4. a) Vegetable soup with 2 pieces of plain bread or 2 Indian chapatis; b) 2 fresh tomatoes.
5. The same as in the preceding days.

Seventh day:

1. The same as in the preceding days.
2. The same.
3. a) 1 glass of fresh juice (any); b) 1 bowl of fresh vegetable soup
4. a) Vegetable fresh soup with 2 pieces of plain bread or 2 Indian chapattis; b) 2 slices of cottage cheese with a piece of plain bread.
5. The same as in the preceding days.

Eighth day:

1. The same as in the preceding days.
2. The same as in the preceding days.

3. The same as in the preceding days.
4. The same as in the preceding days.
5. 1 glass of boiled warm or cleaned water with lime and honey.

Ninth day:

1. The same as in the preceding 5th or 8th day.
2. The same as in the preceding days.
3. a) 1 glass of fresh juice; b) 1 bowl of fresh soup (any); c) 1 bowl of lightly cooked vegetables.
4. The same as in the 6th day.
5. The same as in the 1st and 7th days.

Tenth day:

1. The same as in the 1st day.
2. The same.
3. The same.
4. The same.
5. The same.

Notes:

1. No salt and no sugar should be used in the food.
2. Onion and garlic must be used very sparingly.
3. Obesity people must take 1 glass of juice or tea at one taking; others may take those 2 at once, but slowly sipping.
4. Never take food hurriedly! Instead chew it well and then swallow little by little. It is very important!!!
5. Take first water, tea, juice, soup, then pass on to the chewing of your food. Never take them together! All liquids must be chewed as well!

It's difficult to live like this, but if you appreciate your health and your well-being, you must and must live like this only.

6

YOGA IS LIGHT

It is the celestial light divinely ordained,
It is the wisdom of ages which yogis obtained,
It is for the betterment of humanity,
It is health and prosperity,
It is to keep away the ills of body and soul from posterity.

(Courtesy—Sidh Parkash Kaushik.
Haryana (India)
June 25, 1990. Dushanbe.)

It is nonsense saying that illness is one's fate and there is no case for one to live a short period of lifetime.

Do you know what life is? I don't think that you can answer this question totally right. I may answer it all truthfully this way. Life is a play, and that's all. As a rule every play has rules of playing. The same is the case of the play of life. They are well described as Yam and Niyam in Yoga:

1. Non-violence.
2. Sathya—Truth.
3. Asteya—Non-robbery.
4. Aparigraha—non-accumulation of wealth.
5. Brahmcharya—celibacy,
6. Shaucha—clean body.

7. Mittahar—Limited vegetarian food.
8. Santosha—satisfaction of anything.
9. Swadhyaya—getting much knowledge.
10. Tapas—ascetism.
11. Ishwarapranithana—Total surrender to God.

One who follows these rules of life; he achieves and wins the game for excellence. But alas! Most of the people aren't able to understand why they are living on earth, what is their real task among people or why are they human being at all.

As far as we are concerned, we may say that by training physical and spiritual bodies by our way of Yoga, one may become absolutely healthy, strong and young again even if one has lost them already.

I myself am the true example at the age of 80. I don't feel my age as 80, but feel just like 20 or so, though I look somewhat old in appearance as such. Sometimes I feel myself a robot, a machine as I don't feel tiredness while working hard physically or mentally for long. My head is no longer bald. It is as normal with sufficient hair as when I was young. My former weak eyes have turned to be normal. My teeth with hollows are normalized. I have no more tooth arrangement and tooth trouble. I am as flexible as gymnasts and even more. I've no more troubles of any disease as it happened some 20 years ago;—I was then a bucket of all diseases. By 50 years of age I felt myself as old as 80 and was afraid of dying soon.

By following our way of Yoga teaching many Tojikistonians have been returned to normal way of life, to work. Physically disabled have become strong again and returned to their former work,

These are the chronicle diseases we heal up: arthritis, gangrene, epilepsy, bronchial asthma, diabetes; lung, heart, kidney, spleen, pancreas, stomach ulcer, small intestines, large intestine, rectum, duodenum, enteritis, rheumatics and many other diseases of human body.

To propagate our method of healing diseases by our Yoga way of life, we use the large scale of publicity through newspapers and journals, magazines, radio, television and we publish books.

Here is then a paradox:

Everybody wants to live healthy and long, and nobody wants to be old soon. However, when one offers them what they desire, they just don't believe. Moreover, they don't want to help you any way, financially or otherwise.

The well known Russian writer N. Ostrovski said: "Man's dearest possession is life and he must live it so as to feel no suffering, regrets for wasted years and never know the burning shame of a mean and petty past. So while dying he might say: "All my life, all my strength was given for the finest cause—the fight for freedom of all the Mankind".

It was uttered in the early years of 20th century. Now I'd like to reiterate the same most willingly and add this:

"All my life, all my strength I will give for the fight of freedom of all the Mankind to come out of the bondages of ailments and vices of life. It is my highest dream, the Essence of my Life travel!"

Until one is not healthy physically he is not healthy spiritually too. The better the Health the finer the spirit will be there in the body. It brings us to the conclusion like this:

The more the society is healthy the more the Country is Wealthy. The more the people are rich in spirit the more the Country prospers.

From this point of view, I call upon you, readers and all the people of the World to 'raise arms against the sea of' diseases and 'by opposing fight' against and "end" them for the welfare of humanity! I call yogis, gurus, saints, sages, doctors and medical workers all over in the world!

I BEG YOUR PARDON, OH, IMMORTAL PEOPLE OF THE WORLD! DO YOUR BEST NOW FOR YOUR SELF AND FOR THE SAKE OF THE FUTURE PROSPERITY OF MANKIND!!!

7

YOU ARE NO "FOOLS"

0h, yes, I'm not mistaken. Let me prove, my opinion in "black and white" words. Please do not get offended. Let me be fully frank and tell you the whole truth.

Let me open your eyes wide on the reality of life and your being human being on Earth. If you find my words hard or cursing, you don't mind and don't take it seriously for blaming. I'm writing it all for bringing a drastic change, to amaze you and remind you that there is something more, unusual awaiting you. I simply love you, and want to do things for your good, that's all.

Let us look around at things seriously, attentively, profoundly and find out who we are. From this point of view you must answer one of my startling and the most important question:

—Are you a human being?

I know that everybody answers 'Yes', but I may prove and say that you are only saying "No".

You may find me rough or anything like that, but it is more of a habit, an upbringing, or "culture" of life not to say the truth, because it is bitter. Anyhow I'll try not to hide anything and say everything as it exactly is by nature.

You are becoming fool and rough day by day just by forgetting who you really are. If you call yourself a human being, then tell me, please, why do you kill others, beat, curse, scold and think ill of others? Why do you get angry and aggressive at your surroundings, at the art, the sculpture you've created yourself? Let us look at our characters beginning with our family. Why don't we settle everything here peacefully? At work, how do we behave among colleagues, heads? Can't we settle all misunderstandings positively without scandals? It goes and widens with the borders of the countries, which brings in aggressions and killing all around. Why to kill innocent schoolchildren, steal them, torture them?

Why not make the whole world ONE WORLD without borders? Now tell me, why? Is it normal to fight and kill? Is it a normal human behaviour and the character?

Day by day, "scientists", are producing disastrous machines and guns for so much bloodshed on earth. How they slaughter desperately innocent people using them! Why can't they be aware of their humane heart when killing, beating, and talking ill with somebody or thinking bad about somebody?

Let me remind you who you indeed are and what is the fundamental, most important purpose of your life on Earth?

From Sanskrit Vedic Literature and perennial Indian Philosophy of life we learn that Man has come to be evolved absolutely pure, with no emotion of violence, aggression, hatred, etc. He has got one mission only: to evolve Himself further and become a Superhuman, a God-Man.

From the historical sketches of Bharat we learn that there were about two million of such Supermen and one was living in India till 2012 (Sathya Sai Baba), whom everybody could see and talk, and touch, and 'taste', i.e. I have the experience of being with this True Super human myself.

Having so many super humans among us, all the people of the world, must get experience of them and do things like they have instructed. First of all Indians should be proud, because they have got all chances to be super human faster, living nearer to them. Indian Godman was Swami Sathya Sai Baba in Puttaparthy who was showering LOVE among peoples of the world for more than half century. He was really one whose lifespan should be studied, experienced and followed by everyone all over the world.

All the scientists of the world should do research on Him and others like him. They make everyone on Earth as happy as ever. Looking for subtler knowledge scientists of the world from ancient time till now are mistaken while creating rockets and missiles, bombs and satellites, etc. for killing the living one's only! They are in the jungle of misunderstanding. Even flying to other planets, cannot be a happier choice if we use weapons for killing, even an insect living along on earth. There must be one weapon only—the weapon of Happiness and Prosperity of Mankind:

8

LOVE, LOVE, AND LOVE

"Love is not love which alters when it alteration finds" (Shakespeare).

Now all non-vegetarian people of the world are on the wrong track, on the track of violence and they can never change their minds until they change their food into purely vegetarian kind. It is as true as you are reading this book and thinking I'm telling lie or nonsense. But you are mistaken again as you are used to think, act so.

Killing someone one cannot make his mind to understand the simplest cosmic principle that he'll be killed himself by someone else sooner or later and he can't live like that any farther; he will never be happy indeed! A killer will be killed only.

Let all non-vegetarian eaters know well that they have turned themselves into animals, beasts because their body is fed by animal flesh which is dead and turns mostly into a waste in the body, increasing toxins here and there and calling diseases. Such people will never be happy and will never bring happiness to others, and will live a very short span of life on earth.

Thus, if you do harm to somebody else, you are a fool because Human being is a human being when he does nothing wrong to others and lives in accordance with the Cosmic Law of HUMANITY. This Law is widely explained in Yogic Literature under the titles: YAM-NIYAM, which is practically taught by all gurus, sages and saints all over the world. It is called the Yoga system or the Yogic way of life.

PART THREE

1

IT IS INDIA

Mark Twain in his book "One more trip abroad" (1897) wrote:

"It is really India! It is a dream land of romances, fantastic richness and incredible poverty, significance and rays, palaces and hovels, hunger and plague, giant jinks and Alladin lamps, tigers and elephants, cobra snakes and jungles. It is the country of hundreds of nations and languages, thousands of religious and two million gods, the cradle of human race, the birthplace of human language, mother of history, grandmother of legends, grand-grandmother of Traditions, whose yesterday goes back basically into ancient of all nations.

It is the real country under the Sun allotted to a strange prince and a peasant, educated and narrow-minded, wise and fool, rich and poor, bounded and free. It is the land which everybody wants to see and having seen it only once, even catching a glimpse, one doesn't want to see the other part of the world".

Oh yes, he is absolutely right. When I went there for the first time in 1991, I started wishing to go there again and again and indeed I went there practically every year. Till now I've been there 10 times, and every time it is a new dream for me, just fine and wonderful. I find it like my Motherland. I see in every Indian the image of my close relative.

My dear readers! Born Tojik in the rural mountainous village, in the family of illiterate peasants and living now in the city capital of the Republic of Tojikiston, I find myself almost to be a Hindu and that's why for about 28 years I have been carrying out the propagation of Hindu way of life in a Muslim dominant country of tojiks. Here I propagate the Yoga and vegetarian way of life. I've definitely learned that it is the best and the brightest way of living in the world. Such way of life is the 'sanatan'—the eternal and the original way known to the first man born in the beginning of the history of Mankind on Earth.

It is the Universal Truth which must be understood by everybody. All those who have healthy brain may be optimistic and be with us, but the pessimist is never able to find and understand the same Truth we follow every day.

Thus, I call all Indians and everybody in the world, who are optimists to be more active for carrying out their duties more sincerely, for which one must learn and bring up oneself in accordance with Yogic Yam—Niyam laws of life.

The greatness of India one may simply learn by understanding and following God-Man Sai Baba who is well known and followed all over the world. One may learn Him by his books, literature, messages recorded all over the world. Secondly, the greatness of India is also its visual beauty. All over India there are so many historical monuments, castles and temples which remind the most skilled and architectural divinity of people existing there. There are so many sages and saints, gurus who give the education of spirituality and divinity in the ashrams and Yoga centres which is spread everywhere in India.

Physically, even by shape and form it is like the heart of the world. Being continuously fed by pious water of rivers like Gangaes, Narmada Brahmputra etc, like the nerves of the blood, it is as if the nourishing point of the world.

2

INDIA IS INDEED GREAT

Willingly coming to India for many times I don't find myself a stranger here, as its people are most hospitable, generous and respectful. Why not! Historically, Indians are certainly the most peace loving people in the world.

Now I am fully convinced that India is the cradle of Human civilization. It is the heart capital of the whole world because everyone living on earth looks towards India with the hope of getting a spark of divinity as here were many avatars (incarnations) of Divine personalities. Even now one was completing His mission successfully till 2012. He was Bhagwan Shri Sathya Sai Baba in Puttapartty.

Baba was great and He was making India well-known all over the world. He was turning it into the Centre of utmost knowledge, divinity and humanity. He was 'inviting' peoples of the whole world to His ashrams, schools, colleges, institutes and universities. His Super Speciality Hospital in Puttparthy and other hospitals are serving needy ones free of charge from anywhere in the world. He has explained the meaning of the word "Hindu" letter by letter. It is like this:

> H stands for HUMANITY.
> I stands for INDIVIDUALITY.
> N stands for NATIONALITY.
> D stands for DIVINITY.
> U stands for UNITY.

Here we see all the best characteristics of a man. It means that an Indian is a real HINDU when all the 5 above mentioned qualities are present in him/her. Of all these,—said Baba,—'HUMILITY' is also very important.

Thus, in Puttapartty and White Field Ashrams in Banglore thousands of peoples from the whole world gathered and became staunch devotees of Sai Baba. Baba was bringing them up to change their way of life, i.e. get rid of bad habits and tendencies and become vegetarians, serve others as gods and love every one on earth.

I became a vegetarian in 1990 when I had understood the significance of it after reading the book "Bhagavad-Gita" and profoundly started following the philosophy of Yoga. Since then I'm feeling myself better and better, younger and younger as I go in for Yoga seriously.

Here, I have many highly respected friends who are all vegetarians and they are helping me to understand things and matters rather practically. To name out of them a few, they are Mr. O. Baig, Mr. H. S. Greval, Mr. D. Chopra, Mr. L. Vaid, Mr. S. Gupta, etc. who are members of BGP and managing directors of some important companies.

From my point of view, we must study lessons of life from India and try to be like 'HINDU'. India is really the richest and the greatest country in the world. Most of Hindus follow the saying: "Help ever, Hurt never'.' Rightly all true Hindus are vegetarians because being non-vegetarian one cannot be a real Hindu as animal's flesh makes the body full of wastes and illness. Where there is waste and there are the diseases. There is no purity of mind and body in it also.

Being among vegetarian people in India, I feel myself like an Indian, as if it is my Motherland. I don't feel going quickly back home. Here I am among sincere friends, whom I call 'my brothers & sisters'. Here I feel myself as safe and sound as nowhere in the world. After being here for the first time in 1991 I liked to come here again and again. I have no wish to go to any other country, but India.

India is as old as Mankind on Earth. All the knowledge of the world originated here. For the improvement sake at least, one must come here and see it by his/her own eyes.

Even highly educated Hindus do not know who he/she virtually is.

Being not a Hindu, but living like real Hindu, I feel myself as happy as ever. I feel myself as young as a strong boy even at the age of 80. 27 years ago I was a bucket of diseases and as old as 90 years.

Oh, dear Hindus! Be real Hindus. If you can't make yourself happy, healthy and wise as I recommend, come to me or call me. I'll make you one like me instantaneously. I may remove all your diseases and bad moods. Let's all live under the slogan of non-violence and friendship, as members of one family.

Let us be Lucky and prosper all over the world by living like real HINDUS!

3

INDIAN PAPERS

(Whenever I visited India, Indian news papers often wrote about me as I was always moving among people, yogis giving speeches, telling Indians about my experiences of Yoga with our Tojikistonians whom I have cured from all their diseases by Yoga methods. Being among Indians I had to answer many questions on how difficult is to teach Yoga to those who are ignorant, far from understanding Yoga in a totally Muslim dominated country. Here are some translated pieces of these publications.)

YOGA RECURS TO THE MEMORY WHEN AFFLICTED OF SERIOUS DISEASES

"When people are afflicted with serious diseases, only then remember Yoga" is the opinion of Shri Abduvahob Muhammad Sobirov, a Yoga Scholar from the U.S.S.R. who is here in Bharata these days to study and understand Yoga.

Shri Sobirov, who himself emulates ancient Yoga philosophy manages Yoga Training Corporation in the Republic of Tojikiston in the U.S.S. R. He also conducts Yoga activities throughout the Soviet Russia. There are about one hundred fifty persons of the age group of 60 to 80 attending his Centre receiving Yoga training as a treatment. He claims to have cured hundreds of ailments in cases whom the doctors had denied any possible cure. He believes Yoga is an easy treatment system that can cure all diseases.

A professor of English in Tojik State University Shri Sobirov's introduction with Yoga is only seven years old. Presently, he is completely associated with the spreading, writing and publishing the knowledge, usefulness and dignity of Yoga. He has also translated many Yoga books into Russian. He collected all Yoga Philosophy by going through the English books on Yoga published in India. Shri Sobirov does not have any degree or diploma of Yoga from any Yoga training Institution. He is also a devotee of Sathya Sai Baba. He says, "I am very happy on my visit to India. I feel as if I am among my relatives here. Wherever I go I am very much loved and respected. I have learned very much here". Expressing his knowledge on Yoga he tells, "It is a must for a Yogi to be vegetarian. He must keep away from any kind of intoxication". He says that uncontrolled mind is black, and sugar and salt are white poisons. He is of opinion that without the Government help it is not possible to spread Yoga treatment system. He wants that India and Russia should jointly spread Yoga throughout the world.

Earlier, additional Registrar of the Department of Cooperation, Shri P. D. Mishra, who accompanied the Soviet Yoga erudite, told that during his visit to the U.S.S.R. in 1989, he got acquainted with Shri Sobirov and was profoundly impressed with his authority on Yoga and desired eagerly his visit to India.

The head of the Department of the Yoga training Centre Shri Girish Chandra Khare says that Shri Sobirov shall be conferred with an honorary Diploma of the Yoga Institution.

(Courtesy, MP Bhopal, Nai Dunya, August 6, 1991)

YOGA 1S CAPABLE OF TREATING INCURABLE DISEASES—SOBIR

Minister for cooperation, Government of MP and Soviet Yoga erudite Abduvahob Sobirov made a visit to the Madhya Pradesh Government Yoga Training Centre here. Both of them also blessed the occasion by addressing a gathering of Yoga enthusiasts at a programme.

President of Tojikiston Yoga Association "Iroda" Dushanbe, U.S.S.R Shri Abduvahob Muhammad Sobirov said that Yoga has been presently recognized as a Medical system of treatment. Yoga has been proved as a sure cure of certain incurable diseases. Mr. Sobirov told that many big cities in different provinces and republics of the U.S.S.R. now have Yoga training centres where people reach in large number. He said that Yoga is, now, an internationally recognized developed system.

The Cooperation Minister Shri L. N. Sharma narrating the dignity and importance of Yoga said that he shall extend all help to the Government Yoga Training Centre, Bhopal. On this occasion presenting a report on the Centre, Shri Girish Chandra Khare, Head of the Department, told that by making arrangements at the District headquarters of the State, this year, about three thousand teachers have been imparted the Yoga Training through about two hundred Yoga Resource persons.

Shri P.D. Mishra, Additional Registrar of the Department of Cooperation of the MP State, a Yoga enthusiast, who accompanied Shri Sobirov also addressed the meeting. On this occasion, the Yoga Instructors of the Centre Shri Agnihotri, Smt. Saroj Pandey and Shri Yadava demonstrated some Yoga asanas.

The head of the Department of the Training Centre Shri Girish Chandra says that Shri Sobir shall be conferred with an honorary Diploma of the Yoga Institution.

(Courtesy, MP Bhopal, Danik Bhasker, July 26, 1991.)

GOVERNOR FOR EXPANSION OF THE YOGA EDUCATION

BHOFAL: Noted Russian Yoga Master Mr. Abduvahob Muhammad Sobirov demonstrated the different Yoga postures at a simple function organized at Raj Bhavan. He also delivered a lecture on benefits of Yoga. The Governor, Kunvar Mahmud Ali Khan, described his demonstration as a unique example of Indian Yoga Darshan. Minister for cooperation, Mr. L. N. Sharma presided over the function organized by the Government Yoga Kendra. Mrs. Bilkis Mahmud, Raj Bhavan officials and distinguished invitees attended the function.

Speaking on the occasion, the Governor highlighted the importance of Yoga and said that the demonstration of the Russian Yoga exponent testifies to the fact that the people in other countries are increasingly taking to Yoga to make their lives happier and healthier. He, however, stressed the need for further expansion of Yoga education.

Earlier, Mr. Sobirov spoke about popularity of Yoga in the Soviet Union. Mr. Sobirov runs an institution named Tojik Yoga Association in Dushanbe city. He shared his experiences and revealed that earlier he was afflicted with many diseases but the practices of Yoga have cured all these and he is now in the pink of health. His baldness has vanished and he has discarded his spectacles.

(Courtesy, CHRONICLE, BHOPAL, August 27, 1991)

YOGA; THE ONLY WAY TO ATTAIN PEACE, SAYS S0BIR

Only Yoga can help in curing diseases except "Karma" and it is the only way to attain happiness and peace. These words were expressed by Mr. Abduvahob Sobirov, President of Tojikiston Yoga Association "Eroda" while talking to MP "Chronicle" here on Tuesday.

Earlier while replying to a question as to how he got acquainted with Yoga he said that he developed interest in Yoga while he was in the Kazak Republic as Professor of English. He came in touch with another professor who introduced him to Yoga. Since then Yoga had become much a part of his life, he added.

He later practiced Yoga under the guidance of his colleague and books on Yoga.

Referring to Yoga he said it is helpful in curing several complicated diseases. He said that when he took to Yoga he was crippled with large diseases such as blood pressure and heart related problems, but with regular practice of Yoga asans he had been able to overcome these problems. Later he set up an institute at his native city Dushanbe, Tojikiston which started getting good response from the local people there.

While talking about the functioning of the centre run by him he said initially fewer number of people turned up, but he was successful in getting many of them cured of their illness. With success more and more people joined him. Later it was in 1989 when Mr. P. D. Mishra visited the Republic he actually came to learn about the Indian yogis.

Recounting some of his experience, he said that recently a 67 year old man who was suffering from a severe heart attack had joined his institute. He lost all hopes from life, but with the practice of Yoga he started all his normal routine as a healthy person. Similarly in January another girl in her sixteen came to him who was asked by the doctors to go for imputing her leg as it was week. But with the practice of Yoga under Sobirov she has started walking. He attributes his success to regular practice and faith.

Mr. Sobirov said that he ever wished to be in India and learn more about Yoga and meet the learned people to discuss about Yoga at length. He was invited to India by Shri Swami Shivam Tirth of Dewas (MP) whom he later met at Dahisar village Ashram near Bombay recently. He had been to Delhi, Bangalore. He said that with Swami Shivom Tirth he discussed about exchanging representatives from his centre here and vice versa. About India and Indians he said it is one of the most fabulous and celebrated places in the world. He widely appreciated the people who had been very warm and hospitable throughout his stay here.

He said that the best way to be fit was to live on vegetarian food and practice Yoga. He called upon the people to make Yoga a part of their life and live through Yoga.

(Courtesy, CHRONICLE, BHOPAL, AUGUST 28, 1991)

GOVERNOR FELICITATES SOBIROV

BHOPAL: The Governor, Kunvar Mahmud Ali Khan, felicitated Russian Yoga Master, Mr. Abduvahob Mohammad Sobirov, here on Friday at the Raj Bhavan. The governor presented him a shawl, a coconut and books on Yoga. The Secretary to the Governor, Mr. S. K. Mishra, Head of the department of Yoga Centre, Mr. G. C. Khare and other officers were also present on the ocasion.

Mr. Abduvahob, a resident of Dushanbe city of Tojikiston Republic of the USSR, has been in India for the last 40 days. He spent most of the time in exchanging views on Yoga teaching at the Government Yoga Centre in Bhopal. He had demonstrated various exercises of Yoga at Raj Bhavan on August 27 and this was his second meeting with the Governor before leaving Bhopal. Mr. Sobirov informed that he is leaving for New Delhi tomorrow where he will participate in the international Yoga conference to be held from September 5 to 8 and 10th national Yoga Championship. He will go back to Russia on September 18.

Once in 1990 I wrote a letter to the Indian papers. It got published in a number of papers. It is reproduced below:

(Courtesy, CRONICLE, BHOPAL, AUGUST 31, 1991.)

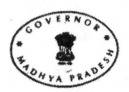

RAJ BHAVAN
BHOPAL-462003

August 30, 1991

I had great pleasure in meeting you at Bhopal and was deeply impressed by your interest in Yoga. From the discussions we had and the demonstration you gave before me, I am quite convinced that you have fully imbibed the spirit of Yoga.

I sincerely wish you all success in your mission to propagate Yoga in your country.

Yours sincerely,

(Kunwar Mahmud Ali Khan)

Mr. Abdubahob Muhammad Sobir,
President of Tojikiston
 Yoga Association,
734036, 265 pos. 40-let,
Oktober, Dushanbe,
Tojikiston of USSR.

4

TOJIK YOGI APPEALS

(PD Mishra got this letter published in some leading papers in India in 1991)

Dear readers in India!

I am writing you from Dushanbe, the Capital of the Tojik Republic. I am Abduvahob Sobirov, 1934, May the Ist. I was born in the northeast part of Tojikiston, in the mountainous valley Bobodarkhon by name. From my childhood I dreamed to be a highly educated person. My parents were illiterate and there was no one literate except the school teachers there who were not also highly educated. They had no full secondary school education. Now, on the contrary, all are literate, highly educated except the very old ones. I was the first and am the only scientist of philology in this rural part of our Republic.

My dreams, step by step, came true. I finished the 7 grade form of local school, then the secondary 10 grade school far from my village- 8 kilometres walking distance on every week-end. There was no transport at that -, time. Then I graduated from the foreign languages faculty the English Department of the Pedagogical Institute in Leninabad town 110 km far from my village. I graduated from it with excellent diploma. It was

1958. I was asked and left at the same faculty as a teacher of English. Then I was in Egypt as an interpreter for six months.

In 1968 I decided to continue my study and entered the post graduate course which I completed successfully in 1973 and became an assistant professor of philology. Thus, up till 2004 I was skilling my grade in this field.

But I was not satisfied with all my successes at all. I was seeking some more urgent, significant in life and couldn't have made clear what that was. It was a secret to me.

All the time 1 was thinking over the problem of life and death. "What for such successes in such a short period of life-time with so many diseases in the body of a man?"—I thought and asked myself very often. I couldn't make clear why a person is born and dies living for so short period of time.

By 50 years of age many diseases tortured me and I became as sick as an old man of 80 waiting for his last period of life on earth. To get rid of my diseases I went in for sport and hard physical culture but they were not of much help for my health. I drank medicine after medicine, tablet after tablets, for long periods of time spent in hospitals . . . It couldn't satisfy me of course.

There was and is one more problem for me, the global problem, with which I am also not satisfied up till now. It is the wanting peace, the obstacles of boundaries, guns and military armies among countries and nations all over the world. I can't understand why a man kills a man or harms each other, why it is not possible to 1ive peacefully, loving each other?

All these dissatisfactions, my dear readers, brought me to YOGA, to "The Bhagavad Gita" as it is, to Krishna Consciousness. Here I've found all the answers I needed. Now I am absolutely satisfied with life itself as I am no longer sick. I am a pure vegetarian now. It is not only me, but the whole family of mine. I have five children: three sons and two daughters (one was expired). We are all Yogis now except my wife. She is not with us yet, because she has the lowest education and doesn't understand yet what Yoga is as those many that doesn't follow it even in your country.

Now during 28 years of Yoga friendship I don't get ill any more. I've got rid of all my diseases I had before. I've become young once again. I've turned into a robot-like man as I never get tired while working physically or mentally from early morning till late at night. I've forgotten what is a headache or sore throat or lung diseases, heart attacks, legs and back troubling. I couldn't read or write without a looking glass anything. Now I am writing this letter without it.

You see, I was a bald man. Now I am not. My head is full of hair again. I'm seeking now to have them all black, but I have a little experience as yet, I think.

I had teeth troubling since 1960. Now they are just no disturbing me, but have grown to full. I've forgotten where the dentist's clinics are. Now I've forgotten where the road to medical services' offices is.

On having learned and found such a truth and happiness in Yoga system I couldn't help being silent and thus organized a little centre /cooperative/ of Yoga in Dushanbe city, the capital of Tojikiston in September 13, 1988, In march—June of 1989 appeared in our centre Prabhu Dayal Mishra, a yogi from Bhopal, India. He highly appreciated my beginnings in Yoga path and published his opinions here in Dushanbe papers and there in India. You might have read them and learned all about.

Now I have turned this little cooperative into an Association of Yoga in the whole of Tojik Republic. It is going to be a much larger centre of Yoga here. I am the President of it till now.

In October of 1989 /19-21/ the fist Yoga Congress took place in Moscow, where I took an active part. There gathered many yogis from all parts of the Soviet Union. There were representatives of Yoga centres from 15 countries abroad. There came from your country, India, Shri B.K.S. Iyengar, the well-known Guru all over the world. On the scene of yoga training, among all the yogis gathered there Iyengar tested me and appreciated highly. We together were photographed and placed in "Moscovskaya Pravda" newspaper on October the 21st, 1989. There an American Yogi presented me a thick book "Yoga for everyday life" saying: "It had been offered by the author for you . . ."

So I had chats almost with all the Yogis from other countries. Retuning to Byelorussia's capital city Minsk where 1 had been skilling my scientific doctorate work and it had to be finished at the end of 1989, I began fasting and successfully had to break it in 10 days.

There in Minsk I met Krishna servants and made close contacts with them so that I invited them to Dushanbe. They did agree and then I had them here under the head of their general director Mamu Thakur das.

Sick people who came to me, though they were glad and satisfied with my Yoga training, I was not satisfied myself as I had very little experience on Yoga and had not been in any school of Yoga anywhere. I wasn't in India either . . . .

Oh, great, great Gurujis! Help me, please to become as great as you are. Invite me, officially, arrange my coming to your Yoga centre and let me have a close contact with True Yoga visually.

May be some Yoga center will take over my yoga center in Dushanbe under its guide and will direct our Yoga activity both spiritually and materially?

For present time I have some contact with your people who come here for study and cooperative exchange activity. It is P. D. Mishra from Bhopal, the excellent friend. This year in April there came some more among whom are Mr. K. S. Kashep,

Mr. R. H. Sinkh, Mr. S. P. Kaushik. They are helping me in preliminary Yoga matters as they are not professional ones.

Now I have a great, great dream: through Yoga to connect all the people of the Republic of firstly Tojikiston, and then the other countries of the world, particularly India and Tojikiston.

Sincerely Yours, A. M. SOBIROV.

My address: 734036, 265, Navruz Street, Dushanbe, Tojikiston.

5

TOJIK YOGA ACHARYA

(- I came across YOGA in 1984 by chance. Since that time I am learning it from its bottom to its top continuously through books and peoples life. I am going through Yoga not only by learning it theoretically, but by practically using it in my everyday life and just not alone, but along the whole people of the Republic of Tojikiston.)

In 1988 He set up an official, cofirmed by the Minister of Justice of our Republic, Association, i. e. "Tojikiston Yoga Association "'IRODA". Now it is well known all over the world, especially in India. Coming to Yoga Motherland very often for the purpose of learning and experiencing much about Yoga, He has come to the conclusion that India, this land of ancient past, is as miraculous as the natural YOGA itself, i. e. Astanga YOGA.

After He came to India in 1991 for the first time, He couldn't stop coming here again and again. He does not have even any wish to visit any other country in the world, but India. Why? Because He has found here the precious treasure, i.e. the treasure of happiness—youthfulness in the old age and long healthy life—the Truth of life.

Having seen and travelled from North to South, from East to West, in India, He has made a discovery: India is the HEART, CRADLE, and the CAPITAL of the World. Look at its shape on the Map,—it's like Heart, surrounded by water like the blood veins around it, and historically all the countries of the World have been originating their culture, knowledge and science from its treasure store—Vedas.

About India and Yoga He tells;

-Dear Indians, I may demonstrate a set of miraculous, disease curing, vice removing asanas at the age of 80, when I am as healthy, strong and flexible again as I was at the age of 20, like a sportsman or a gymnast. You know when I was under the age of 50 I was as old as 80 or more and as sick enough as a helpless old man. I was bald-headed with a looking glass, sick heart, teeth troubling and many other misfortunes of unhealthy body with a bouquet of non-curable diseases. Now they are all removed off from my body. It is because of my changing the way of life into yogic, Indian, vegetarian way of life. Mind that only pure vegetarian way of life is the best one.

You may be absolutely sure that I've told you the Truth, the Cosmic Truth.

Oh, Indians, you may be proud of the fact that you are Indians as you are really living on this Holy Land. You've got all the opportunities here to be as great as the God Himself, say, like Swami Sathya Sai Baba in Puttaparthy or like many other saints and sages here who are the wisest men on Earth.

Thus, there is an unchangeable Truth which one must follow in the span of one's whole life. It is:—Do everything Right, say everything Right, live on Right path as it is written in "The Gita". In that case only you'll achieve all the goals of your life.

You never forget that you are living in the most fabulous and celebrated place of the world. India is as great as the Heaven as such! Take your chance easily, don't hesitate, go in for Yoga every day, and follow my advice if you want to be as happy as I am at this old age.

If I were you, oh, my dear Indians, I should have done things around much better than you are doing them now.

Dear Indian Yogis, let us make peoples of the world understand what is what by our moving and "fighting" because: 'Alive must fight, and alive are only those whose hearts are given to the highest goal', told Victor Hugo. And this goal I have found in YOGA only. Truly, only Yoga can assure the Happiest, the Healthiest and the Longest span of Life on earth!

(A summation of some other stories appearing in Indian papers)

PART FOUR

1

WE ARE MEMBERS OF ONE FAMILY

We have come today to the most Fabulous and Celebrated Place in the world!

Historically and geographically India must be supposed to be the Capital of the whole world. Why not! In ancient times because of its spiritual leadership India gave the Message of Peace to the World. Then as well as now, the Bharattiya Message has been like this:

"Let all the people everywhere be Happy"!

We may very well say that the best universal knowledge originates here in India. That is why we are here very often to see and tell you the unique Truth and who you really are.

Oh, my dear Indians! You are just unaware of the significance of being HINDUS and how really you matter to the whole world. But we, Tojikistonians, know it. That is why we are here very often, in India. We'd like to see the Divine and divinity here by our own eyes and get more experiences of divinity from you.

There in Tojikiston learning the knowledge of Yoga by books only and experiencing it for about 27 years, putting it into practice among the citizens of our country I have come to the conclusion that it is the most attractive philosophy and the best way of life. It is the medicine of all the diseases. Moreover, it is the cheapest way of life, through which one becomes not only strong, but gets cured of all diseases both physically and mentally without any medicine. Vegetarian food is the only right food suggested by God for Human Being. It is never costly.

Humanity means harmony in thought, word and deed. Today this harmony is totally lacking.

How should, one live? One should live in accordance with the upanishadic prayer which says:

"Let us grow together, live together in one accord and develop.".

Man today is unable to understand what life is, what its goal is, what one's duty is and what one's aim should be. Time is moving fast like a whirlwind. Man's allotted span of life is melting every moment like a block of ice. Man's life ends even before he is aware of his duty.

What is duty?

Every individual has some aspirations, some ideals to be realized and some sacred paths to be trodden. But he makes no effort to pursue these aims.

What is the goal and purpose of one's life? What are his secrets?

Man hardly puts these questions to himself. He is contented in devoting himself to sensuous pleasures. This is not what he should do. It is not the aim of life.

Everything is based on man's thoughts, which finds expression in external forms as a reflection of his inner being. Thoughts lead to action. There can be no action without thoughts. It is essential to entertain sacred thoughts. Everyone should realize that all the sorrows and miseries of modern man are due to his evil thoughts. Every man thinks that someone else is responsible for his troubles. This is not so. We alone are responsible for the good and evil that befalls us. We blame others because of our weakness.

Thoughts, words and actions should be in harmony. This is the mark of a true human being. This basic truth is valid without regard to place, nationality, language or religion. It is applicable to people everywhere, at all times. Those who observe this triple purity are redeemed. They are the salt of the earth. They are the upholder of righteousness.

Man today should reflect on his true nature. The Lord declares in "THE GITA":

"The individual on earth is a fragment of my Eternal Self".

'The import of this declaration is:

"Oh man! Don't think you are only a composite of the five elements. You are a fragment (Amsa) of me".

A branch is a part of a tree. A child is a part of the mother. The branch cannot survive without the tree. The child cannot survive without the mother. Man is a fragment of Madhava (the Supreme Self). Hence man cannot exist without Madhava. But, it may be asked: "Is man not surviving today? How is he doing that?" But what kind of life is he leading? Is he living, as a human being? No! He is living as an animal. If he were aware that he is a spark of the Divine, why is he a prey to suffering?

In Sai Baba's words we may conclude the followings'

—Does Cod have any worries or troubles? None at all. He is in eternal bliss, bestowing all happiness, and the embodiment of all wisdom. If you are a fragment of that Divine why should you be a prey to all this sufferings? When you enquire in this manner you will realize that you are not behaving like a spark of the Divine.

You must take a pledge from today to lead a godly life. The man without love is lost in dialectical controversies; with the result of the bitterness in argumentation erupting.

Human beings have come to the planet Earth as pilgrims. They have to return to their original homes. You have come from Parmatma. You have to go back to the Parmatma. You have come from the Brahman (Supreme Self). You have to merge in the Brahman. You have incarnated as a spark of Brahman. You have to become the Brahman. That is the ideal. That is the goal. In between there may be many impediments. You should ignore them. Have unshakable faith. That is the true devotion for all.

2

YOGA IS A GLOBAL CULT

1. Yoga is self realization above all.
2. Yoga is unity with Allah, secondly.
3. Yoga is freedom, thirdly.
4. Yoga is peace, fourthly.
5. Yoga is Love, fifthly.
6. Yoga is an ever youthfulness, sixthly.
7. Yoga is a healthy way of life, seventhly.
8. Yoga is longevity, eighthly.
9. Yoga is Happiness permanent, ninthly.
10. Yoga is oneness all around, with the people of the world and with the Universe, tenthly.
11. Yoga is total well-being, the eleventh.
12. Yoga is the life—breath, the twelfth.
13. Yoga is wholeness with Nature, the thirteenth.
14. YOGA IS the ESSENCE OF Supreme God, ALLAH—ALLAH'S BODY, WORDS, BREATHS, SOUL, and MIND AND BRAIN. IT IS HIS reflection and the shadow.
15. GOD IS IN YOGA & YOGA IS IN GOD!
16. Yoga is well-being of a man forever.
17. One who doesn't understand it he is really ignorant & despicable!
18. Who wishes being despicable? Will you tell me, who?
19. You see, no one!
20. Then why waste time?

21. YOGA IS A METHOD BY WHICH ONE CAN DEVELOP ONE'S INHERENT POWER IN A BALANCED MANNER. IT OFFERS THE MEANS TO REACH COMPLETE REALIZATION. THE LITERAL MEANING OF THE SANSKRIT WORD YOGA IS 'YOK' ACCORDINGLY. YOGA CAN BE DEFINED AS A MEANS FOR UNITING THE INDIVIDUAL SPIRIT WITH THE UNIVERSAL SPIRIT OF GOD.
22. YOGA IS WELL-BEING, ABSOLUTE HEALTH AND LONGEVITY

3

THE SMILE OF YOGIS

Smile is pleasure of mine and yours.
Smile is light of sights of our hearts.
Smile, and Smile, where's yours?
Smile is the key of all hearts.
Stop! My friend, friends so dear,
Young and old, people of the Earth!
Where's your May Day Smile,
Healer of the burning of the Planet?
Without Smile there won't come wealth,
As in the body of a patient—health.
Without Smile life on Earth's impossible,
To work, to create, to make wonders!
Stop! Smile, where's the Smile of yours,—
Healer of the wound of your soul?
Where's a celebratory Smile of yours,—
The Elixir of pleasure and my dream?
Smile the workers of the whole Planet,
Forge iron cheerfully at the machine tools!
To live on Earth's impossible without Smile
To work, to create, to make wonders!
Stop! The Smile, where's your Smile?
Address me & others with nice Smile,—
Friendship begins with a Smile too,
With a Smile a cloudy day is bright.

Smile the soldiers of the universe!
Throw guns and automatic devices!
With Smile you'll be safer and safer!
On the Planet from the threat of war!
Stop! My friend, friends and dear,
Young and old, people of the Earth!
Where's the warm Smile of yours,—
This reliable coat of our Planet?
Listen oh, people, the people of the Earth!
Live with peace, friendship and smile.
You see the friendship begins with Smile.
Sleep with Smile and wake up with Smile!
Stop! The passer-by, drivers and pilots,
The people of the whole universe!
Show me the true Smile of yours,—
Smile with me—all boys & girls!
The smile is peace, love and friendship!
The smile is the key for all your doors!
The native Land begins with your Smile!
Stop! My friend, friends and dear mothers,
Young and old, people of the Earth!
Teach your child to Smile from birth.
Children of yours from dawn to dawn!
Listen the people, people of the Earth!
The Earth of ours, you see, round,
And our purpose should be uniform.
Let it be uniformed, there'll be Smile!
Smile the Man of the planet, the Earth!
Smile and do not hesitate anymore!
Without Smile the life is impossible,
To work, to create, and to make wonders!
The workers of countries incorporate!
To the Smile of uniformed be ready!
Smile with me and do not hesitate,
Smile and be always well & healthy!
It is me, the Yogi Yogishwranand SOBIR.
It is me, the Youth of the world.
Lighted up by Great Consciousness,
Born by the Smile of the Founder.

I call you, Youth of the World,
I call you, all the peoples of the world,—
Of any colours Mankind of the Earth,
Be ready; to smile be always ready!
The people of the world of any colours.
It is me, the eternally young Yoga,
Eternally green, but mature Yoga.
Living long, long years with Smile,
Five thousand years have I lived.

*   *   *

4

TOJIKISTON YOGA ASSOCIATION "IRODA"

Under a heading "Photo reporting" the edition of the newspaper "Dushanbe Evening" brought out with photos under the caption "There is a Yoga Association of Tojikiston!", where the following is printed:

-This day in the Palace of culture of trade unions the fans (amateurs) and professionals of Yoga were gathered. They have gathered in Dushanbe from all ends of the Republic to discuss a question on establishment of Yoga Association of Tojikiston. Officially there has arrived from Moscow the president of Yoga Association of the USSR L. I. Teternikov.

The conference was opened by the vice-president of Tojik RS (VDFSO) of Trade Unions V. V. Kovinev. Marking a weak condition of businesses on improvement of the population of the republic, he welcomed voluntary and noble undertaking of yogis of the Republic. Having noted thus, that RS (VDFSO) of Trade Unions acts in this case as the first founder—sponsor, he has expressed a wish, that other organizations engaged in improvement of the population health should have also followed this path.

Then president of Yoga Association of the USSR, L. I. Teternikov shortly stopped on principles of work of the Association. Supporting the creation of Yoga Association of Tojikiston, he has assured that the all-Union organization will render all assistance to its activity.

The member of the Presidium of the Council of Yoga Association of the USSR, chairman of medicinal-improving cooperative society "IRODA" on Yoga system, senior lecturer of Tojik Pedagogical Institute of Russian language and literature by A. S. Pushkin, A. M. Sobir acquainted the participants of the conference with the ethics of Indian Yoga.

The statement of the worker of the Tojik TV Mirzo Davlatov was interesting also. With Yoga he has got acquainted with the cooperative Yoga society "IRODA" and under the direction of its chairman A. M. Sobir, more than two months were engaged hardly. In such a short term he got rid of serious diseases, which oppressed him since long time, and in their treatment medicine did not help. Moreover, he has reset (dumped) superfluous weight. Regular running in the mornings could not help any more.

Pondering on the philosophy-psychological aspects of Yoga, the senior scientific employee of the department of philosophy of Tojikiston Academy of sciences Muhammad Ali Muzaffar, in detail has deciphered all eight steps of Hath-Yoga, without which the development of the man cannot take place for becoming a true yogi.

"In my life Yoga has played a magical role",—so the teacher of the English language Flora Abuzarova began the statement. Being engaged the whole year, she has not only got rid of illnesses, but also has found out in herself (as also in her daughter, Lola) abilities of the psychic power.

The participants of the conference have accepted the Charter of Yoga Association of Tojikiston. In it, in particular, it is written down, that «the Yoga Association of Tojikiston is a public organization uniting the separate persons and any organizations of the republic, engaged in Yoga or promoting to its development". Its purpose and tasks are the creation and development of a network of organizations, organisation of scientific—practical conferences, symposiums, seminars, study of impact of Yoga practice on the man, development of the improving programs, training of the Yoga teachers, establishment of communications (connections) with the foreign Yoga centres, and publishing papers and books.

The President of Yoga Association of Tojikiston unanimously elected is A. M. Sobir, Vice-President M. Muzaffar and executive secretary F. Abuzarova.

5

RECLAMATION OF YOGA

"Man's dearest POSSESSION is Life
And he must live it so
As to feel no tortures, regrets
For wasted years never unknown
The burning shame of a man
Of the petty past". (N. Ostrovski)
YOGA> MAN > YOGA

YOGA IS A GOD'S COMPOSITE IDEA. Since the appearance of the first Man on Earth God wanted the Man not to suffer, not get ill and not to die sooner, but to live a long and happy life. For this purpose God provided Man both the theory and the practice of Yoga which we call Yoga philosophy.

God wished the Man while developing morally to turn himself into His image and just suffer not. It's necessary to begin with Love for everything around in Nature with nonviolence, without harming anyone alive by word, deed and even by thought. At the same time one should not forget that God is like this Himself. Man gets ill and suffers because he does not carry out the God's instructions in performing his own duties in life. For not fulfilling his responsibilities enshrined by God, man gets punishment not from God, as some think, but from himself, his own nature. All mistakes and errors of Man are large writ in his subtle body—in the black box.

THERE'S NO OTHER WAY! THERE'S NO OTHER WAY! THERE'S
NO OTHER WAY!

Remember the cycle!
MAN>YOGA>GOD
PROGRESSING EVER

6

SOME PUBLICATIONS BY P.D. MISHRA AND COURTESY EXTRACTS

Yoga co-operative Tajikistan

(i) AN ERA BEGINS

(**The author P.D. Mishra, the leader of Indian Delegation of Cooperative Management Training in Cooperative Institute Dushanbe wrote this article which was published in 'Communist Tajikistan' Dushanbey in April,1989. Courtesy**)

I will call it a very pleasant surprise to find a "Yoga Cooperative" working in Dushanbe in the guidance of a dedicated teacher Abdul Wahab Sobir. I had read in the Indian News Papers, that people in USSR are increasingly taking interest in Indian Yoga system but I could not believe my hostel warden suddenly pronounce 'Yoga' when she noticed me meditate in my room.

It is also difficult to believe that the ENT specialist of a hospital introduced one of my colleagues to Abdul Wahab for his health problem since her medical and surgical treatment would not suit him much.

This is a timely recognition of an ancient science by a rational society of a highly developed country like USSR. I am sure due to the second great revolution taking place under PERESTROIKA in the USSR its cultural and spiritual ties with India shall be further strengthened by a closer cooperation of the two peoples systematic investigation into a hitherto many unknown secrets of YOGA.

While interviewing these practitioners of Yoga in the centre, I have been asked some very important questions about the background of Yoga and different modern schools of its working in India. I therefore herein intend to impart some information about this science of India.

Yoga is one of the six systems of Indian philosophy. Through these systems or theories of philosophy, Indian seers of the past have tried to explain the purpose of life, world and the overall design of God or nature. Yoga lays greater stress on human capabilities. According to this theory it is not important whether there is God or not but there undoubtedly exists such a higher potential in a human being that he can reach the heights of Godhood of Man's belief and conception. The founder of this science was PATANJALI whose theory has been propounded in his famous work 'YOGA DARSHAN' (the science of yoga). Yoga Darshan explains in detail that there are eight steps of yoga progress.

These are Yama (mental restraint), NIYAMA (Adherence to certain rules). ASHAN {Physical postures), PRANAYAMA (breathing exercises), PRATYAHAR (making mind introspective), DHYAN (meditation), DHARNA (contemplation), and SAMADHI (realisation of truth), In brief, physical and mental preparation is necessary for one to tread the higher paths of YOGA.

Another famous exponent of Yoga system is Lord Krishna. Krishna's classical conversation with his friend and disciple Arjuna is recorded in a unique book called 'Gita'. Krishna does not so much talk about philosophy in it since Arjuna is facing a mighty army in the battlefield and he must have an immediate and practical solutions about his doubts whether it is proper for him to kill his close relatives, ill directed against him though, in the battle field or not. In essence, Krishna first argues that every living being has an immortal and mortal part of his existence and to believe one to be dead is to mistake the fact. For Arjuna, he points out, that when a man becomes Yogi his actions are 'Karma Yoga' (Actions of Yoga), in such actions there is necessarily an added **efficiency** and they thus do not have a binding effect of future cause and action.

This science of Yoga long remained confined to the monks and mendicants for centuries and it is also a noticeable feature of modern age of new science that the intellectual class of modern society all over the world is so much attracted towards it. Tilak and Mahatma Gandhi were perhaps first modern Indians who put this knowledge into practice for the liberation movement of India, In 1893 Swami Vivekanand startled the world by demonstrating the splendor of Yoga after his participation in the conference, on World religions in Chicago (USA). His teachings on Rajyoga are immensely popular ever since and there are numerous institutions run after his teachings of Yoga and they are doing many constructive services of the society in India and abroad.

Broadly, Yoga in India has two main branches. Hath Yoga (Yoga of physical exercises) and Dhayn Yoga (the Yoga of meditation). The manipulation like Bhakti Yoga (The Yoga of devotion), Karm Yoga (the Yoga of Action), Gyan Yoga (The Yoga of knowledge), and Rajyoga (the Yoga of superior knowledge), all come under the second category. The former has been widely incorporated in the educational system of India and the State owned media like Television has a regular weekly program for about half an hour owing to its practical significance for the physical fitness of the people. The Yoga of meditation is a system of mental experience of expanding consciousness and enjoys a high social recognition. I have accompanied myself Maharashi Mahesh yogi thrice in All India Institute of Medical Sciences, New Delhi when experiments about the efficacy of his transcendental meditation were going on as early as in 1968-69. According to this system, the meditation effectively releases people from every day's stress and strain and fills them with **an** added energy, intelligence and happiness after meditation.

An absolutely authentic record of the splendor of Yoga is available in the Biography of Yoganand Paramhan's book called 'An Autobiography of a Yogi". This Yogi died in 1952 and his dead body was certified by eminent **physicians to** be intact and undecayed even after 24 days of his death. We find the firsthand record of this yogi describing how he met his teacher Yukteswar in Regent Hotel Bombay at 3 pm on 6th June, 1939 after 99 days of the physical expiry of his guru. He had a 3 long hours' discussion with him while receiving advance courses on this science further. He has given in it a photograph of Mahaavtar Baba also who was his great grand teacher and who according to him was living for more than 3500 years.

Late Shri Shivanand Saraswati of Rishikesh UP, India himself a doctor initially, made immense contribution towards a systematic exposition of this science through many books on the subject and has a wide ranging following in India and abroad. His organization is known as "Divine Life Society" and after his expiry is headed at present by highly enlightened and scholarly teachers Chindanand and Krishanand.

Yoga tends to become a mystical science in course of the expansion of consciousness of a man. Yogis tell that there is a mysterious power called Kundalini at present lying dormant at the base of spinal cord in every human being. If this energy is awakened and activated, a man can perform miracles by effecting conscious control on his autonomous nervous system. He can also at the same time experience extra sensory perceptions like hearing, seeing and smelling things at any distance or time. Some Yogis call it the system of Shaktipat (The incidence or fall of energy from the enlightened on to the disciple). By following this system, the aspirant does not have himself to take any trouble of effort fully doing the physical exercises because they occur automatically once the dormant power of the person is awakened and put to action. Late Swami Vishnuteerth of Dewas (MP) India (his disciple, and the present Swami Shivom Teerth does have this competence now). Late Swami Muktanand of Bombay and Acharya Rajnish at Poona may be referred to fall in this category.

At the level of devotional aspect, the properties of Yoga have been vitalized by Bhaktivedant Prabhupad of Krishna Consciousness and Sai Baba of South India. Shrila Prabhupad prescribes a Mantra for chanting whose sound vibrations take such a person on a transcendental plane. Sai Baba is a man of miracles. He says that miracles are as much inherent in his nature as much as the normal physical movements are in the nature of any ordinary human being. I have myself witnessed a number of miracles while visiting him thrice in his place and also several times from the distance of thousands of kilometers. I have seen many kilograms' sacred ashes falling from his empty hand and the materialization of many precious objects from nowhere. The greatest of all his miracles is the universal love flowing from his person which keeps about many million peoples of the world in his following. His Yogic presence is felt and experienced by thousands of people all over the world.

I am sure this movement in Tajikistan in particular and the USSR in general shall soon gain ground and people shall be immensely benefited by it.

*   *   *

(ii) SAI BABA IN TAJIKISTAN

By P. D. Mishra

Tajikistan, a republic of the erstwhile USSR now an independent nation of Russian Common-wealth is fast coming in the fold of the following of Shri Satya Sai Baba of Puttapartty (South India). This is evident from a number of letters received by me from Abduvahob Sobirov who visited India in the late summer of 1991. Abduvahob has accompanied me to Puttapartty for Sai Baba's darshan there. I very well remember Abduvahob with a large card in his hand inviting Sai Baba in his direction with the inscription "from the USSR". This is a practice among devotees there that since they do not have full chance to talking to Baba and seek his blessings to solve their problem; their letters in envelopes are normally taken by Baba while moving among them. This gesture on Baba's part makes devotees believe that their problems have been solved. Thus they normally feel free from the burden they have been carrying.

Abduvahob was just disappointed when he could not get this chance sitting in forward rows after standing for hours in long queue for more than half a dozen times there. He was wondering all the time while way back for what should have been the reason of it. We were normally sitting together at such time, but it so happened on our day of departure that Baba walked much closer towards me and while I could seek his blessings as desired, Abduvahob remained far away.

Nevertheless, Abduvahob purchased all such article which would remind him of Baba's grace and presence anywhere. I have been since receiving all sort of articles which Abduvahob is publishing in his country about his experiences and his visit to Puttapartty in search of knowledge. Abduvahob was basically a yogi teaching yoga exercises which he had picked up from a few books available in his country. It was difficult for him to find a teacher and find books on the subject with every possible detail. He had therefore followed me to India for practicing Yoga rigorously here. Abduvahob writes that since prices have gone very high in his country due to collapse of the Soviet Power, people are now opting for Yoga for curing their diseases as it involves no money or medicine. It is a very simple reason as it might appear, but Abduvahob and people have now come to believe in the divinity of a living God, Sai Baba in his country. He is constantly writing, lecturing and appearing in television and radio broadcast in propagation of super natural powers and the universal love manifested in one personality—Sai Baba. Abduvahob has also written that he is under practical guidance and supervision of Sai Baba in every step he takes and every move he makes in his life. He has thus been able to achieve whatever he has been striving for.

It's not to be concluded that people should start believing in miracles. Sai Baba never teaches that. Whatever miracles are seen or performed by him are not owing to any effort made on his part since they are as integral part of his nature as any natural movement of us. His message can be summed up in one word that is "Love", a universal love, divine love, a living bond among mankind. It is only out of love towards humanity that Baba wants to emancipate human beings here by providing better schemes and colleges for true education, hospitals for better medical facilities and selfless services, to human society. May be, this story opens up many shut eyes in India about a true light of knowledge emanating from a living divine presence—Sai Baba.

Published in National Mail, (daily) Bhopal August 11 1995 (paper courtesy)

*　　*　　*

(iii) TOJIK YOGA TEACHER IN CITY

Tojik Yoga teacher Abduvahob Sobirov demonstrating techniques at the Government Yoga Training Centre in the City on Tuesday. HT Correspondent *Bhopal, March 23*

YOGA PRACTITIONER and teacher from Tojikiston, Abduvahob Sobirov today demonstrated Yoga techniques At the Government Yoga Training Centre and told Participants that **yoga** could help keep away all kinds of **ailments.** Interestingly, Sobirov has himself received training from the Yoga centre here. On this occasion, Sobirov put on a badge of Tojikiston on Yogacharya Miss Pandey of the Government Yoga Training Centre. His son Alisher also demonstrated yogas to cure stomach ailments. Sobirov is also a professor of English and a great yoga enthusiast. He answered various queries of the people who attended the session, Pt K. P. Agnihotri, Mangesh Yadav and O. P. Shrivastava welcomed him at the outset. A number of bureaucrats and senior citizens attended the programme.

(Courtesy—**HT Bhopal Live**, Wednesday, March 24. 2004)

*   *   *

(iv) RUSSIAN YOGA TEACHER HAS SHOWN KRIYA YOGA

Abdul Vahob Sobir, the Yoga teacher from the republic of Tajikistan of Russian Federation has shown today here before the citizens, how Yoga can benefit ailing people. Shri Sobirov has told, that Yoga can cure all illnesses of the man. 70-years old Sobirov does not show any of the attributes of the old age in him. He has informed that his body is very flexible, as he practices Yoga each day. Earlier he had received educational experiences at the state Yoga Centre in Bhopal. He has given gifts to the teachers of the Centre. They were the badges with the image of Yoga asans. He has given them in a mark of friendship and memoirs. He has expressed the pleasure of meeting with the old friends strongly by embracing them.

*   *   *

(v) REAL PEACE WILL COME

The scientist on Yoga system Abduvahob Muhammad Sobirov in the country of Tojikiston is engaged in Yoga with the citizens and has arrived in India to exchange experience and to train Indians on advanced Yoga system. He has learnt Yoga from the books independently and has got full theoretical knowledge after combining it with practice by him. In 1990 he had arrived in Bhopal at the invitation of PD Mishra and had then exchanged experience at the state Yoga Centre. He told about it in a meeting with the chief editor of the newspaper "Nirdaliy"(Neutral) Kailash Admi. At the meeting also there was present an associate of the newspaper a doctor Ramgulam Bitsha "Raghu". Mister Sobirov has this time arrived in India at the invitation of the state Centre of health and Ministry of health on March 9, 2004 in New Delhi and on March 21 took part in the release of the book of the well known writer in Delhi.

Since 1990 he has come to India 9 times. First time he came at the invitation of Shri Prabhu Dayal Mishra whom he met in Tojikiston in 1989, when he went there on an official trip as the head of a delegation of Government workers.

Mister Sobirov has informed the gathered audience in the hall that he has published more than 100 articles and 10 books about Yoga in Tojikiston. His books are titled: "The Art to live hundreds of years and be Healthy", "Each man can become the Superman ", "Secrets of Guru", "Rich health" written in the Tojik and Russian languages, which became very popular there. He has also published the book under the title "Yoga and keys of health for youthfulness and longevity ". When asked, how being a Moslem he was interested in Indian Yoga, mister Sobirov answered, that Allah (God) is one for all. He is equally kind and great for everyone.

Despite the progress of science and engineering in modern times, Sobirov believes fully in God, though he is a teacher of the English language in his country. He had incidentally found a Yoga teacher while teaching English language in Kazakhstan in Pavlodar town while working together with a Russian gentleman in the college of Pavlodar. This teacher provided mister Sobir the book of Dhirendra Brahmachari "The Science of Yoga", in which he got engrossed instantly and later engaged himself in Yoga thoroughly and also studied it independently. He has also said further that in that time he had pains in a backbone with heart ailment. But when he began to engage himself regularly in Yoga, gradually his illnesses disappeared and now he is completely a healthy man. Mister Sobirov has also asserted that he can concentrate on Yoga practices all the 24 hours a day and just not forgetting it even for a minute.

(An extract from the story published in "Nirdaliy" weekly, Bhopal in 2004 with courtesy)

*　　*　　*

APPENDIX

TABLE OF CALORIE RECKONER

We reproduce here (with our acknowledgment due to Dietary Department of Indraprasth, Apollo Hospital, New Delhi) "Calorie reckoned" after shortening and changing them suitably from the point of view of the vegetarian way of life. Having followed this table one will really understand the importance of edible portion of raw food products, and will surely change his way of life for better.

a) VALUES ARE GIVEN PER 100 GM OF RAW FOOD'S EDIBLE PORTION

S. No 1	Name of foodstuff 2	Fat gm 3	Protein gm 4	Carbohydrate gm 5	Energy K.Cal. 6
1.	Amla	0.1	0.5	13.7	58
2.	Apple	0.5	0.2	13.4	59
3.	Apricots (fresh)	0.3	1.0	11.6	53
4.	Apricots (dried)	0.7	1.6	73.4	306
5.	Avocado pear	22.8	1.7	0.8	215
6.	Bael fruit	0.3	1.8	31.8	137
7.	Banana (ripe)	0.3	1.2	27.2	116
8.	Blackberry	0.5	1.3	6.7	37

9.	Bread fruit	0.2	1.5	15.8	71
10.	Cashew fruit	0.1	0.2	12.3	51
11.	Cherry (red)	0.5	1.1	13.8	64
12.	Currants (black)	0.5	2.7	75.2	216
13.	Dates (dried)	0.4	2.5	74.8	317
14.	Dates (fresh)	0.4	1.2	33.8	144
15.	Figs	0.2	1.3	7.6	37
16.	Grapes (blue variety)	0.4	0.6	13.1	58
17.	Grapes (pale green variety)	0.3	0.5	16.5	71
18.	Grape fruit (Marsh's seedless)	0.1	1.0	10.0	45
19.	Grape fruit (Trumph)	0.1	0.7	7.0	32
20.	Guava (country)	0.3	0.9	11.2	51
21.	Jack fruit	0.1	1.9	19.8	88
22.	Lemon	0.9	1.0	11.1	57
23.	Lemon (sweet)	0.3	0.7	7.3	35
24.	Lichi	0.2	1.1	13.6	61
25.	Lime	0.1	1.5	10.9	59
26.	Lime (sweet, Malta)	0.2	0.7	7.8	36
27.	Lime (sweet, Musambi)	0.3	0.8	0.3	43
28.	Mango (ripe)	0.4	0.6	16.9	74
29.	Mangosteen	0.1	0.5	14.3	60
30.	Melon (musk)	0.2	0.3	1.5	17
31.	Melon (water)	0.2	0.2	3.3	16
32.	Mullberry	0.4	1.1	10.3	49
33.	Neem fruit	1.0	1.3	15.1	75
34.	Orange	0.2	0.7	10.9	48

35.	Orange Juce	0.1	0.2	1.9	9
36.	Papaya (ripe)	0.1	0.6	7.2	32
37.	Passion fruit	0.1	0.9	12.4	54
38.	Peaches	0.3	1.2	10.5	50
39.	Pears	0.2	0.6	11.9	52
40.	Phalsa	0.9	1.3	14.7	72
41.	Pine apple	0.1	0.4	10.8	46
42.	Plum	0.5	0.7	11.1	52
43.	Pomegranate	0.1	1.6	14.5	65
44.	Prunes	0.3	0.5	12.8	56
45.	Rasins	0.3	1.8	74.6	308
46.	Raspberry	0.6	1.0	11.7	56
47.	Sapota	1.1	0.7	21.4	98
48.	Seethaphal	0.4	1.6	23.5	104
49.	Strawberry	0.2	0.7	9.8	44
50.	Tomato (ripe)	0.2	0.9	3.6	20
51.	Wood apple	3.7	7.1	18.1	134

b) VEGETABLES

1	2	3	4	5	6
1.	Banana rhizome	0.2	0.4	11.8	51
2.	Beef root	0.1	1.7	8.8	43
3.	Carrot	0.2	0.9	10.6	48
4.	Colocasia	0.1	3.0	21.1	97
5.	Lotus root	0.1	1.7	11.3	53
6.	Mango ginger	0.7	1.1	10.5	53
7.	Onion (big)	0.1	1.2	11.1	50
8.	Onion (small)	0.1	1.8	12.6	59
9.	Parsnip	0.3	1.3	23.2	101
10.	Potato	0.1	0.6	22.6	97
11.	Radish (pink)	0.3	0.6	6.8	32

12.	Radish (rat-tailed)	0.3	1.3	4.3	25
13.	Radish (white)	0.1	0.7	3.4	17
14.	Sweet potato	0.3	1.2	28.2	120
15.	Tapioca	0.2	0.7	38.1	157
16.	Tapioca chips (dried)	0.3	1.3	82.6	338
17.	Turnip	0.2	0.5	6.2	29
18.	Yam (elephant)	0.1	1.2	18.4	79
19.	Yam (ordinary)	0.1	1.4	26.0	111

c) LEAFY VEGETABLES

1	2	3	4	5	6
1.	Amaranth (tender)	0.5	4.0	6.1	45
2.	Aralkeerai	0.4	2.8	7.4	44
3.	Bamboo (tender shoots)	0.5	3.9	5.7	43
4.	Bathua leaves	0.4	3.7	2.9	30
5.	Brussels sprouts	0.5	4.7	7.1	52
6.	Cabbage	0.1	1.8	4.6	27
7.	Caelery leaves	0.6	6.3	1.6	37
8.	Colombo keeral	0.4	2.5	3.7	28
9.	Colocasia leaves (black variety)	2.0	6.8	8.1	77
10.	Same (green variety)	1.5	3.9	6.8	56
11.	Coriander leaves	0.6	3.3	6.3	44
12.	Curry leaves	1.0	6.1	18.7	108
13.	Drumstick leaves	1.7	6.7	12.5	92
14.	Fenugreek leaves	0.9	4.4	6.0	49
15.	Knol-khol greens	0.4	3.5	6.4	43
16.	Kappa Keera	0.3	5.2	3.8	38
17.	Kuppameni	1.4	6,7	6.0	64
18.	Lettuce	0.3	2.1	2.5	21
19.	Manal Keera	0.4	2.4	2.3	22
20.	Manathakkali leaves	1.0	5.9	8.9	68

21.	Mini	0.6	4.8	5.8	48
22.	Mustard leaves	0.6	4.0	3.2	34
23.	Neem leaves (tender)	3.0	11.6	21.2	158
24.	Parsly	1.0	5.9	13.5	89
25.	Paruppu Keera	0.6	2.4	2.9	27
26.	Pasarai Keera	0.4	1.7	7.9	42
27.	Poonanganni	0.7	5.0	11.6	73
28.	Puliara Keera	1.5	4.3	7.2	60
29.	Radish leaves	0.4	3.8	2.4	28
30.	Siru Keera	0.3	2.8	4.8	33
31.	Spinach	0.7	2.0	2.9	26
32.	Tables radish leaves	0.6	3.9	4.2	38
33.	Velai Keera	0.8	6.5	8.8	68

d) OTHER VEGETABLES

1	2	3	4	5	6
1.	Agathi flowers	0.5	1.0	4.4	26
2.	Artichoke	0.1	3.6	16.0	79
3.	Ash gourd	0.1	0.4	1.9	10
4.	Beans (scarlet rubber)	1.0	7.4	29.8	158
5.	Bitter gourd	o.2	1.6	4.2	25
6.	Same (small)	1.0	2.1	10.6	60
7.	Bottle grourd	0.1	0.2	2.5	12
8.	Brinjal	0.3	1.4	4.0	24
9.	Broad beans	0.1	4.5	7.2	48
10.	Cauliflower	0.4	2.6	4.0	30
11.	Celery stalks	0.1	0.8	3.5	18
12.	Cho-Cho-marrow	0.1	0.7	5.7	27
13.	Cluster beans	0.4	3.2	10.8	16
14.	Colocacia stem	0.3	0.3	3.6	18
15.	Cawpea pods	0.2	3.5	8.1	48

16	Cucumber	0.1	0.4	2.5	13
17.	Double beans	0.3	8.3	12.3	85
18.	Drumstick	0.1	2.5	3.7	26
19.	Drumstick flowers	0.8	3.6	7.1	50
20.	Figs (red)	0.6	1.2	10.8	53
21.	Field beans	0.7	3.8	6.7	48
22.	French beans	0.1	1.7	4.5	26
23.	Giant chillies (capsicum)	0.3	1.3	4.3	24
24.	Jack (tender)	0.3	2.6	9.4	51
25.	Kandan kathiri	0.8	3.1	4.8	39
26.	Karonda (fresh)	2.9	1.1	2.9	42
27.	Kovai	0.1	1.2	3.1	18
28.	Knol-khol	0.2	1.1	3.8	21
29.	Ladies fingers	0.2	1.9	6.4	35
30	Leeks	0.1	1.8	17.2	77
31.	Lotus (stem dry)	1.3	4.1	51.4	234
32.	Mango (green)	0.1	0.7	10.1	44
33.	Papaya (green)	0.2	0.7	5.7	27
34.	Peas (green)	0.1	7.2	15.9	93
35.	Pink beans	0.4	3.1	7.0	44
36.	Plantain flower	0.7	1.7	5.1	34
37.	Plantain green	0.2	1.4	14	64
38.	Plantain stern	0.1	0.5	9.7	42
39.	Pumpkin fruit	0.1	1.4	4.6	25
40.	Pumpkin flowers	0.8	2.2	5.8	39
41.	Ridge ground	0.1	0.5	3.4	17
42.	Snake ground	0.3	0.5	3.3	18
43.	Sword beans	0.2	2.7	7.8	44
44.	Sandafi (dry)	1.7	8.3	55.0	269
45.	Tinda (tender)	0.2	1.4	3.4	21
46.	Tomato (green)	0.1	0.9	3.6	23
47.	Vegetable marrow	0.1	0.5	3.5	17

e) CEREAL AND PRODUCTS

1	2	3	4	5	6
1.	Bajra	5.0	11.6	67.5	361
2.	Barley	1.3	11.5	69.6	336
3.	Jawar	1.9	10.4	72.6	349
4.	Maize (dry)	3.6	11.1	66.2	342
5.	Same (tender)	0.9	4.7	24.6	121
6.	Oatmeal	7.6	13.6	62.8	274
7.	Raji	1.3	7.3	72.0	328
8.	Rice (parboiled, hand pounded)	0.6	8.5	77.4	349
9.	Same (parboiled, milled)	0.4	6.4	79.0	347
10.	Same (raw, milled)	0.5	6.8	78.2	345
11.	Same (raw hand pounded)	1.0	7.5	76.7	346
12.	Rice flakes	1.2	6.6	77.3	346
13.	Rice-puffed	0.1	7.5	73.6	325
14.	Semolina	0.8	10.4	74.8	348
15.	Wheat (whole)	1.5	11.8	71.2	346
16.	Wheat (whole)	1.7	12.1	69.4	341
17.	Same (refined)	0.9	11.0	73.9	348

f) PULSES AND LEGUMS

1	2	3	4	5	6
1.	Bengal gram (whole)	5.3	17.1	60.9	360
2.	Same (dhal)	5.6	20.8	59.8	372
3.	Same (roasted)	5.2	22.5	58.1	369
4.	Black gram dhal	1.4	24.0	59.6	347
5.	Cow pea	1.0	24.1	54.5	323
6.	Field bean (dry)	0.8	24.9	60.1	347
7.	Green gram (whole)	1.3	24.0	56.7	334
8.	Horse gram	0.5	22.0	57.2	321

9.	Ehesari dhal	0.6	28.2	56.6	345
10.	Lentil	0.7	25.1	59.0	343
11.	Peas (dry)	1.1	19.7	56.5	315
12.	Same (roasted)	1.4	22.9	58.8	340
13.	Rajmah	1.3	22.9	60.6	346
14.	Redgram dhal	1.7	22.3	57.6	335
15.	Soyabean	19.5	43.2	20.9	432

g) NUTS AND OILSEEDS

1	2	3	4	5	6
1.	Almond	58.9	20.8	10.5	665
2.	Cashew nut	46.9	21.2	22.3	596
3.	Chilgoza	49.3	13.9	29.0	615
4.	Coconut (dry)	60.3	6.8	18.4	662
5.	Same (fresh)	41.6	4.5	13.0	444
6.	Groundnut	40.1	25.3	26.1	567
7.	Same (roasted)	39.8	26.2	26.7	570
8.	Jungle badam	35.5	11.4	—	—
9.	Mustard seeds	39.7	20.0	23.8	541
10.	Pistachio nut	53.5	19.8	16.2	626
11.	Walnut	64.5	15.6	11.0	687

h) CONDIMENTS AND SPICES

1	2	3	4	5	6
1.	Asafoetida	1.1	4.0	67.8	297
2.	Cardamon	2.2	10.2	42.1	229
3.	Chillies (dry)	6.2	15.9	31.6	246
4.	Same (green)	0.6	2.9	3.0	29
5.	Cloves (dry)	8.9	5.2	46.0	286
6.	Coriander	16.1	14.1	21.6	288

7.	Cumin seeds	15.0	18.7	36.6	356
8.	Fenugreek seeds	5.8	26.2	44.1	333
9.	Garlic (dry)	0.1	6.3	29.8	145
10.	Ginger (fresh)	0.9	2.3	12.3	67
11.	Lime peel	o.5	1.8	29.4	129
12.	Mace	24.4	6.5	27.8	437
13.	Nutmeg	36.4	7.5	28.5	472
14.	Omum	21.8	17.1	24.6	363
15.	Pepper (dry)	6.8	11.5	49.2	304
16.	Same (green)	2.7	4.8	13.7	98
17.	Tamarind pulp	0.1	3.1	67.4	283
18.	Turmeric	5.1	6.3	69.4	347

i) MILK AND MILK PRODUCTS

1	2	3	4	5	6
1.	Milk (buffalo's)	6.5	4.3	5.0	117
2.	Same (cow's)	4.1	3.2	4.4	67
3.	Same (human)	3.4	1.1	7.4	65
4.	Curd (cow's milk)	4.0	3.1	3.0	60
5.	Butter milk	1.1	0.8	0.5	15
6.	Skimmed milk (liquid)	0.1	2.5	4.6	29
7.	Channa (cow's milk)	20.8	18.3	1.2	256
8.	Same (buffalo milk)	23.0	13.4	7.9	292
9.	Cheese	25.1	24.1	6.3	348
10.	Khoa (whole buffalo milk)	31.2	14.6	20.5	421
11.	Same (skimmed buffalo milk)	1.6	22.3	25.5	206
12.	Same (whole cow milk)	25.9	20.0	24.9	413
13.	Skimmed milk powder (cow's milk)	0.1	38.0	51.0	357
14.	Whole milk powder (cow's milk)	26.7	25.8	38.0	496

j) FATS AND OILS

1	2	3	4	5	6
1.	Butter	81	-	-	729
2.	Ghee (cow)	100	-	-	900
3.	Same (buffalo)	100	-	-	900
4.	Hydrogenated oil (fortified)	100	-	-	900
5.	Cooking oil (groundnut, custard, coconut, etc.)	100	-	-	900

k) MISCELLANEOUS FOODSTUFFS

1	2	3	4	5	6
1.	Arecanut	4.4	4.9	47.2	249
2.	Arrow root flour	0.1	0.2	83.1	34
3.	Betel leaves	0.8	3.1	6.1	44
4.	Bread (broun)	1.4	8.8	49.0	244
5.	Same white	0.7	7.8	51.9	245
6.	Cane-sugar	0.0	0.1	99.4	298
7.	Coconut (tender)	1.4	0.9	6.3	41
8.	Coconut milk	41.0	3.4	11.9	430
9.	Coconut water	0.1	1.4	4.4	24
10.	Coconut meal (deoiled)	2.8	23.8	47.9	312
11.	Honey	—	0.3	79.5	319
12.	Jaggery (cane)	0.1	0.4	95	383
13.	Same (coconut palm)	0.2	1.0	83.5	340
14.	Same (date palm)	0.3	1.5	86.1	353
15.	Mango powder	7.8	2.8	64.0	337
16.	Mushroom	0.8	3.1	4.3	43
17.	Pappad	0.3	18.8	52.4	288
18.	Pappy seeds	19.3	21.7	36.8	408
19.	Sugar cane juice	0.2	0.1	9.1	39

20.	Toddy (fermented)	0.3	0.1	1.8	38
21.	Same (sweet)	0.3	0.1	14.3	59
22.	Yeast (dried, brewer's)	0.6	39.5	39.1	320
23.	Same (food)	1.8	35.7	46.3	344

SOME YOGA POSTURES

Lying asana of perfection

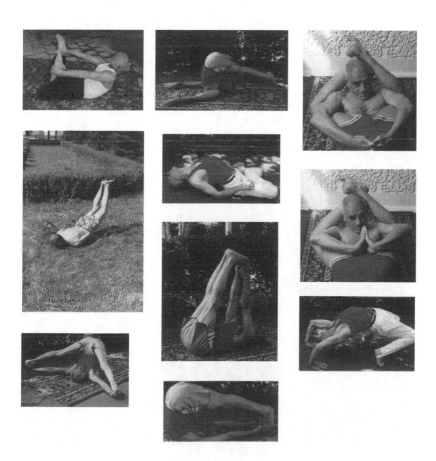

A. Sobirov (Yogishwaranand)

PRABHU DAYAL MISHRA-1946
President Maharshi Agastya Vedic Santhanam, Bhopal, India

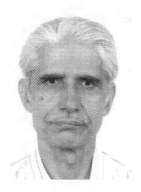

BIRTH—October 16, 1946 in village Barmadang, Tikamgarh.

EDUCATION—M. A. (English) from University of Sagar, M. P., India.

LIVELIHOOD—Retired as senior official of the Government of Madhya Pradesh. Consulting /visiting/ participating academician in universities and various Institutes and organisations.

JOURNEYS—Travelled throughout India along with Maharshi Mahesh Yogi in connection with his Spiritual Regeneration Movement (1968-69), worked as instructor of Hindi and Indian culture in American Peace Corps (1970), Lectured on Gita and Yogadarshan in Tajikistan, Uzbekiston Republics of the erstwhile U. S. S. R. (1989) and United States of America (2004, 2010).

INITIATION—Yoga, Shaktipat and Vedas.

PUBLICATIONS—Saundarya Lahiri, Kavyanuvad—1990. The Gita for All—1994. Sabke Liye Gita—1996. Uttarpath—1998. Maitryi—1999. Veda Ki Kavita—2001. The Holy Vedas for All—2002. Veda Ki Kahaniya—2004. Sab Ke Liye Veda—2006. Tantra drishti Aur Saundarya Shristi—2007. Ishvar Ka Ghar Hai Sansar—2008. Yog Ke Sat Adhyatmic Niyam (translation)—2009. Tantra Drishti and Saundarya Shrishti (second edition)—2012. World: The Abode of God—2013, The Way Farther—2013, Doorva Dal —2013 and Yatra-Antaryatra—2013.

HONOURS—Felicitation in Rashtrapati Bhawan—1994, Vyas Purashkar by The Madhya Pradesh Sanskrit Academy for Saundarya Lahiri, Kavyanuvad in 1997, Felicitation in Madhya Pradesh Rajbhavan for 'Veda Ki Kavita' in 2002, Puskar Award by Madhya Pradesh Lekhak Sangh—2005. Excellence Award by International Penguin House—2006. Mahakavi Keshav Samman—2010. "Pranaam" by Hindi Bhawan, Bhopal—2011.

PRESENT STATUS—President Maharshi Agastya Vedic.

Sansthanam, Bhopal.

CONTACT—35, Eden Garden, Choona Bhatti, Bhopal, MP, 426016.

E-MAIL:—1. pdmishra@operamail.com. 2. vishwatm@hotmail.com

Web- www.vishwatm.com, Facebook- Prabhu Mishra, Blog-prabhu-mishra. blogspot.com